MW01193662

THE GALLBLADDER DIET GUIDE

The Complete Diet Guide for People with Gallbladder Disorders

MONIKA SHAH

Gallbladder Diet, Gallbladder Removal Diet, Gallbladder Flush Techniques, Lifestyle Changes along with Yoga's, Mudras and Home Remedies for fast & Instant Pain Relief

The Gallbladder Diet Guide - The Complete Diet Guide for People with Gallbladder Disorders
Copyright © Monika Shah, 2016

Printed in the United States of America by CreateSpace, On-Demand Publishing, LLC
(An Amazon Company)
www.createspace.com

ISBN-13: 978-15-44174-37-2
ISBN-10: 1544174373

Production Credits
Illustrations by Aaskformore
Cover design by Aaskformore
Text design by Monika Shah
Edited by Monika Shah
Printed by CreateSpace, , On-Demand Publishing, LLC

Disclaimer

The information contained in this book is not designed to replace or take the place of any form of medicine or professional medical advice. The information in this book has been provided for educational and entertainment purposes only.

The information contained in this book has been compiled from sources deemed reliable, and it is accurate to the best of the Author's knowledge; however, the Author cannot guarantee its accuracy and validity and cannot be held liable for any errors or omissions. Changes are periodically made to this book. You must consult your doctor or get professional medical advice before using any of the suggested remedies, techniques, or information in this book.

Upon using the information contained in this book, you agree to hold harmless the Author from and against any damages, costs, and expenses, including any legal fees potentially resulting from the application of any of the information provided by this guide. This disclaimer applies to any damages or injury caused by the use and application, whether directly or indirectly, of any advice or information presented, whether for breach of contract, tort, negligence, personal injury, criminal intent, or under any other cause of action.

You agree to accept all risks of using the information presented inside this book. You need to consult a professional medical practitioner in order to ensure you are both able and healthy enough to participate in this program.

For all those who are suffering with gallbladder problems or disorders.

CONTENTS

UNDERSTANDING YOUR GALLBLADDER   1

THE IMPORTANCE OF THE GALLBLADDER   3
STRUCTURE OF GALLBLADDER   4

THE GALLBLADDER DETERIORATION STAGES AND GALLSTONES   7

STAGES OF DETERIORATION OF GALLBLADDER   7
Stage 1 – Formation of Gallstones   8
Stage 2 – Onset of the Gallbladder Diseases   8
Stage 3 – Further Deterioration   9
GALLSTONES - THE MAIN CULPRITS   10
Gallstones' Formation Workflow   10
The Types of Gallstones   12
Cholesterol Gallstones   12
Black Pigment Gallstones   13
Brown Pigment Gallstones   13
Mixed Gallstones   13
Common Bile Duct Gallstones   13
GALLBLADDER DISORDERS THAT DO NOT INVOLVE GALLSTONES   14
Acalculous Gallbladder Diseases   14

IDENTIFYING GALLBLADDER PROBLEMS   17

THE SYMPTOMS AND STAGES   17
Colic, or Biliary Pain   18
Timeline of Gallstones' Discovery   19
Acute Cholecystitis   19
Chronic Cholecystitis   21
Choledocholithiasis   22

THE MEDICAL DIAGNOSTICS FOR GALLBLADDER RELATED ISSUES   **25**

ELIMINATING OTHER HEALTH CONCERNS   25
PHYSICAL EXAMINATION   26
LABORATORY TESTS   27
IMAGING DIAGNOSTIC METHODS   27
ENDOSCOPIC ULTRASOUND   28
COMPUTER TOMOGRAPHY (CT) SCANS   28
X-RAYS   28
CHOLESCINTIGRAPHY   29
ENDOSCOPIC RETROGRADE CHOLANGIOPANCREATOGRAPHY (ERCP)   29
COMMON MEDICAL TREATMENTS   30

MOST COMMON FACTORS WHICH CAUSE GALLBLADDER RELATED AILMENTS   **33**

LIFE AFTER REMOVAL OF GALLBLADDER   **41**

WHY GALLBLADDER REMOVAL IS REQUIRED?   41
GALLBLADDER SURGERY   44
DOCTORS' ADVICES TO THEIR PATIENTS   44

LIFE HABITS TO PREVENT A GALLBLADDER ATTACK   **47**

FOODS AND HABITS THAT ARE BEST AVOIDED FOR THE GALLBLADDER   **51**

FOODS TO AVOID   52
UNDERSTANDING FATS IN FOOD   59
PLAYING THE HUNGER GAMES RIGHT!   60

FOODS THAT ARE HEALTHY FOR THE GALLBLADDER   **65**

IDEAL MEAL PLAN FOR PEOPLE WITH GALLBLADDER PROBLEMS   **71**

IMMEDIATELY AFTER WAKING UP   71
BREAKFAST   72
MID-MORNING SNACK   72
LUNCH   72
DINNER   72
DIET FORMATTING WITH FIBER   73

NATURAL HOME REMEDIES FOR GALLBLADDER PAIN RELIEF   **75**

REMEDY 1   76
REMEDY 2   76
REMEDY 3   77
REMEDY 4   77

REMEDY 5   78
REMEDY 6   78
REMEDY 7   79
REMEDY 8   79
REMEDY 9   79
REMEDY 10   80
REMEDY 11   80
REMEDY 12   81

**NATURAL THERAPIES AND YOGA POSTURES FOR GALLBLADDER PAIN
RELIEF**   **83**

INSTANT PAIN RELIEF ACUPRESSURE REMEDIES   83
MANIPULATION TO PROMOTE BILE FLOW   89
YOGA AND MUDRAS FOR GALLSTONE PAIN RELIEF   96
   Sarvangasana: The Shoulder Stand   97
   Shalabhasana: The Locust Stand   98
   Dhanurasana: The Bow Stand   99
   Bhujangasana: The Cobra Position   100
   Pachimotasana: The Back-Stretching Pose   101
   Viparitakarani: The Upside Down   102
   Trikonasana: The Triangle Pose   103
MUDRAS   105

NATURAL GALLBLADDER DETOX AND GALLSTONE FLUSH   **107**

METHOD FOR PERFORMING GALLBLADDER FLUSH   109
METHOD FOR PERFORMING DAILY GALLBLADDER FLUSH   111
LIFELONG HOME REMEDIES TO PREVENT GALLSTONES   112
   Remedy 1   112
   Remedy 2   112
   Remedy 3   113
   Remedy 4   113
   Remedy 5   113
DAILY LIFESTYLE CHANGES   114

WRAPPING UP!

A Message for Readers!

Heal & Cure Your Gallbladder Disease with the Right Diet & Management

This book has been specifically designed and written for people who have been suffering from Gallbladder disorders and seriously strive to heal and cure it with the help of a healthy and highly effective homemade diet. Apart from taking medications prescribed by the doctor, it is extremely important to eat the right diet to ease the discomfort caused. The book will also unfold various home remedies (step by step procedures), yoga postures (with illustrations), mudras and Gallbladder flush methods to keep your Gallbladder healthy naturally.

Let's take a closer look on what this book has to offer:

Part A – The Gallbladder Disease Guide

This part of the book educates you not only about the Gallbladder disease itself, but also the causes, symptoms, various stages of Gallbladder deterioration, Gallstones and their various forms, various types of medical diagnostics and all other aspects related to Gallbladder disorders. It also covers in detail about the life after Gallbladder removal and how one can prevent further Gallbladder diseases and attacks by making simple lifestyle changes.

The primary goal of this part of the book is to make sure that you know and understand all about Gallbladder diseases and how to deal with them effectively.

Part B – The Gallbladder Diet Guide

The primary focus of this part of the book is to guide you on what kind of diet and foods you must eat if you have Gallbladder problems (including Gallstones). This section will unfold the real **dietary** and **nutritional requirements with right sources, best foods to eat, foods to avoid** and **guidelines for making the right choices** while selecting your food. This section makes sure that the person who needs to be on Gallbladder diet is well-versed with the required dietary information and guidelines to keep the Gallbladder healthy and live a comfortable life.

Part C – Home Remedies, Yoga's, Mudras and Gallbladder Flush Guide

This part of the book is a must read if you have Gallbladder disorders. Apart from eating right diet, there are several easy to follow home remedies, yoga's and mudras which can be taken and performed for **instant Gallbladder pain relief**. The book covers all these home remedies, yoga's and mudras in great detail along with easy to follow **step by step procedures** and **illustrations** for better understanding.

Later, it also covers easy to perform Gallbladder flush techniques which one can perform either once, weekly or even on daily basis. The Gallbladder flush will keep your Gallbladder clean and fresh as new always.

Introduction

David Eddings in his book "**Pawn of Prophecy**" had written, "*Little jobs require little men, and it's the little jobs that keep a kingdom running.*" This simple statement has a huge impact when you see it in the context of a human body.

Our body is nothing short of a kingdom, with its many organs, tissues, cells, bones, flesh, nerves, and blood. There are a lot of dramas, emotions, processes, and other activities that happen right within our body! Stand in front of a mirror and you can see your hair, face, eyes, body, and feet reflected. A closer look would probably show you your freckles, eyelashes, and nails. While all these have their own importance, the things that we don't see are the heroes that toil without any glory. Organs such as our heart, kidney, lungs, liver, brain, spinal cord, and our skeletal system are the ones that we commonly hear about and pay close attention to. But what about the little soldiers that also form the army? Without the foot soldiers, there wouldn't be any place or importance for the army generals, would there? Similarly, without the organs such as glands and intestines, the heart and the brain cannot survive and also have no importance.

This book talks about one such little soldier – the Gallbladder. Not many realize this but there are several people who suffer from problems related to this small organ, without even knowing about them until things get out of control. Our body does give us warning signals when any part of our body is not working at its optimum level or is afflicted with diseases, but we often fall behind in reading those signals or mistake them for something less serious. Issues with gallbladder are usually mistaken for an upset stomach caused by bad food or a lot of stress, and even several doctors fail to correctly categorize it to be a gallbladder related problem in its early stages.

This book will also focus on the food items that one must eat to maintain a healthy gallbladder, to help heal a gallbladder that has been damaged to some extent, and for those who have suffered from the loss of the organ. Read on to know more about why food plays such an important role in keeping the body healthy and why it should be kept healthy to live a long-lasting and healthy life. Plus, this eBook offers a bonus chapter to its readers; at the end of the book is a diet plan of one week that will list the food you can consume in a balanced way, to lead an active and healthy life.

It is important to know more about this organ, its importance, how it should be maintained, and what the symptoms of problems associated with it are. This is good to know about all this in advance, before it becomes too late to avoid a lot of pain and loss of the organ.

1

Understanding Your Gallbladder

The gallbladder is a small organ that is located just below the liver. It looks like a small sac or pouch that can be either inflated or deflated, depending on the time of the day. Its dimensions and appearance vary from time to time because just prior to a meal time, the gallbladder is enlarged as it is filled with bile juice. It resembles a pear. After a meal and in between meal times, the organ is deflated as it doesn't store any bile juice. Sandwiched between the small intestine and the liver, this organ is a repository for the bile juice which is produced by the liver. The bile juice is transported by the liver into the gallbladder via small ducts, known as the **hepatitis ducts**.

The gallbladder, when prompted by signals emitted by the brain, pushes the bile it stores into the small intestine, also via a different set of ducts, and that's when it gets emptied and deflated. The brain triggers that need to make the organ contract and expand, but the actual message is delivered by a hormone that is known as **cholecystokinin**. At the prompting of this hormone, the gallbladder pumps the bile in the first section of the small intestine, known as the **duodenum**. The small intestine as a whole, with the help of the bile introduced in it, is responsible for digesting the food we consume. The movement of the gallbladder is similar to the air pouch of a blood pressure measuring machine (manometer). It contracts and expands itself repeatedly so that the bile it contains is transferred to the digestive tract via the common bile duct.

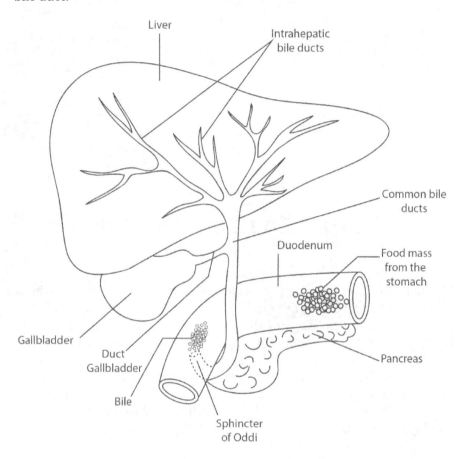

The bile thus transferred is not a simple liquid that just softens food enough to be digested. It performs other functions too. The important ones are:

■ With the help of bile, the intestine is able to emulsify (break down) the fat that is contained in the food and drinks we consume. Once emulsified, the fat can be easily absorbed by other parts of the body to be used as an energy source primarily.

■ Bile is mainly made up of water and bile salts. However, it also contains bilirubin, which is actually the product that is left behind in our body when the hemoglobin in blood is metabolized. Bilirubin can be harmful if left behind in our body and must be eliminated periodically. So bile also facilitates the elimination of bilirubin.

Some of the contents of the bile, such as water and electrolytes, are re-absorbed by the body while it is stored in the gallbladder. This makes bile more concentrated after being stored for some time. That is why the bile that enters the gallbladder and the bile that leaves the organ are not the same. In fact, it is in the gallbladder that most of the fluid content of the bile is extracted every day, and what are left behind are a few tablespoons of concentrated bile. The amount of fluid that is extracted amounts to about 5-6 cups per day.

The gallbladder measures about 3.1 inches in length and about 1.6 inches in diameter. When fully distended, it usually contains about 100 millimeters of bile juice. This small organ is formed mainly of blood vessels and tissues in layers, similar to our skin. It is extremely rare to find a gallbladder that is of a different size or shape; they tend to be the same in almost all human beings. However, there are instances in which the size and shape of the organ have been found to be quite different from the usual standards, and there have been cases reported in which one person has multiple gallbladders, sometimes up to 3 in number. The popular name for this pouch-like organ is gallbladder, but it is also known by other names, such as **cholecyst** and **biliary vesicle**.

THE IMPORTANCE OF THE GALLBLADDER

Unlike the heart and the brain among other organs, it is true that the gallbladder is not a mandatory organ that one must have in order to stay alive and lead a healthy and well-rounded life. However, that doesn't mean that there is absolutely no need to have this organ and that it has zero importance. Elimination of the gallbladder and the possible outcomes of this action have been discussed a little later, but let us first see why the gallbladder is important.

■ The gallbladder is responsible for pumping bile into the small intestine to aid in digestion. It acts on prompts it receives from the brain and performs its duties without which digestion is not a very easy process.

- It acts as a repository for the bile produced by the liver.

- It acts as a store house through which bilirubin can pass through and ultimately be eliminated from the body. So the gallbladder plays a role in keeping the body clean and safe.

- Imagine you have a pan in which you fried a lot of greasy things last night. It wasn't soaked in water and now, the grease has hardened in the pan. When the time comes to wash it off, it becomes a real challenge because of the texture of the grease. Something similar happens in our body when the time comes to absorb the fat from the food and drinks we consume. The body is not equipped to absorb the fat in the form it is in. Nor is the fat available like a cherry atop a slice of cake to be absorbed. With the help of the gallbladder –pumped bile juice, the fat becomes emulsified, only after which the body is easily able to absorb it and put it to use.

- Without bile produced by the gallbladder, some of the nutrition and the good fat, which is necessary for the body to function, will be eliminated from our body while urinating. So the organ may not be mandatory but certainly performs the important task of retaining essential nutrients in our body, unlike any man-made alternative that has been discovered so far.

STRUCTURE OF GALLBLADDER

Nestled between many organs, this hollow organ that has a home in the curve at the bottom of the liver is made up of three segments: the fundus, the body, and the neck.

The point at which the neck of the gallbladder and the cystic duct meet, there is a small pouch or sac that is found, which is a mucosal sac known as the **Hartmann's pouch**. Like many other organs, there are multiple layers of epithelial cells (one of the body cells) that are mainly found in the cavities of organs and as a protective, surrounding membrane around them and blood vessels. This is known as a **mucosal**

layer and the Hartmann's pouch is a mucosal pouch. And it is in this pouch that gallbladder stones are usually found.

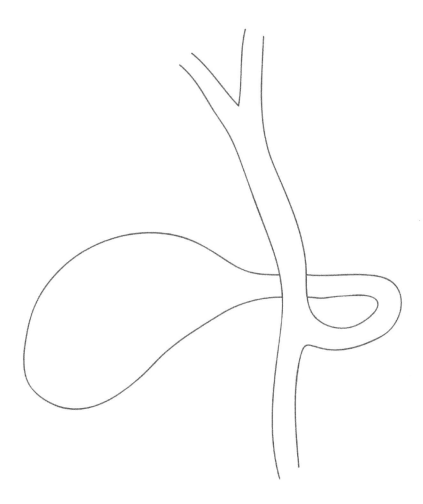

In the next few chapters, there will be discussions about the most important problem associated with the gallbladder – gallstones and the gallbladder areas in which they usually form.

2

The Gallbladder Deterioration Stages and Gallstones

At the right time and the right place, it is good to "have the gall" to perform bold actions! But it is never, ever good to have "gall" stones! There are a few types of issues that can happen to the gallbladder, and they have been discussed in detail in another chapter. But in this chapter, the focus is on gallstones only, and how they impact the gallbladder.

STAGES OF DETERIORATION OF GALLBLADDER

It is said that a known enemy with the fiercest front is better than the foe that creeps up silently behind us and causes us harm. That is because with an enemy who has declared a challenge openly, we know what to expect plus we can think of preventive and counter-attack measures. The silent enemies, on the other hand, are adept in finding our weakest spot and the moment, and choose to attack then. We are caught totally unaware and it becomes too late to be able to fight them off. Gallbladder issues unfortunately belong to the latter category of enemies. Amongst all the health problems that one can suffer from, the breakdown of the gallbladder is one of the most silent and problematic ones. It doesn't mean that people who suffer from gallbladder disorders are suffering from a fatal disease that has no cure. Advanced medical technology is more than equipped to tackle gallbladder related problems. But the discovery of this problem is usually a very painful one. Gallbladder issues that are not treated on time could lead to a rare but more serious problem – gallbladder cancer.

The good news is that there are some indications of gallbladder problems that are easily identifiable by an expert. Recurrence symptoms that are similar to indigestion or stomach upsets should be taken seriously and a physician should immediately be consulted so he or she can check for gallstones. There are other types of illnesses that could impact a gallbladder, but for now, let's look at the three stages in which a gallbladder usually breaks down.

Stage 1 – Formation of Gallstones

The first step in the deterioration of the gallbladder is mostly by the formation of these stones. Gallstones have been discussed in detail a little later in this chapter. They are exactly what they are named as – they are small stones that are made up of bile residues and are of varying sizes. People can have single or multiple small balls that are as tiny as grains of wheat or rice. But some may have gallstones the size of a golf ball too. The really minute stones look like sand particles to the naked eye and can only be recognized for what they are under a microscope. All kinds of gallstones are formed over a period of time and one does not feel any pain or even discomfort when these are being formed. They just remain in the Hatmann's pouch and keep growing in size, while in some people multiple gallstones are formed.

Stage 2 – Onset of the Gallbladder Diseases

In this stage, one starts experiencing symptoms of the gallbladder and the condition deteriorates from time to time. It usually includes abdominal pain, which may be restricted to that area or even spread as far as the upper back. The intensity of the pain, when felt, is quite high and doesn't easily subside even with the release of body gas. The pain however lasts for an hour or sometimes a few hours and then subsides on its own. Some of the other symptoms of this disease are belching, nausea, diarrhea, and burping. These, as we all know, usually happen due to overeating; especially when we consume food cooked using inferior quality oil, meat or other ingredients such as high amount of fat, spices, or sauces.

It is important to note that it is not the formation or presence of the stones themselves that causes these symptoms. It is when the stone or stones start blocking the bile duct (the duct that leads to the small intestine) that the pain and other symptoms are triggered. This is natural because a duct which should be free for normal functioning and thus the body has to find ways to overcome the obstacle or the duct has to be contorted to be able to send the bile juice.

Stage 3 – Further Deterioration

When multiple alarms are missed, or treated as false alarms mistaken for some other common and less dangerous diseases, gallbladder disease enters the third stage. The gallbladder is under immense pressure to transport the bile juice deposited in it regularly by the liver and it is unable to do so because by now, the block either becomes firmer or larger. The stones can increase in number or size (the way the stones are formed differ from person to person and there is fixed way to be able to identify in advance how the stones will be formed in a person, if any) and the gallbladder starts getting inflamed because of the excess of bile juice left in it. The symptoms of this stage are similar to those of stage two, the additional ones being fever, chills, and loss of appetite. But the intensity of the pain increases. Plus, the pain originates from the gallbladder but radiates to a wider circumference in the body. This means that the upper and lower backs could be victim of this pain and the person suffers from discomfort all over.

If a person is suffering from such recurring pain, one must immediately visit a physician rather than taking over-the-counter antacids, digestive aids, or other painkillers. In addition to explaining the symptoms, one must be careful to explain where he/she thinks the pain is radiating from. One easy way to try and differentiate between digestive and gallbladder related pains is that for issues with the latter, the pain will start in the middle of the body towards the right and felt below the liver (which is found in the upper half of the body). The other pains are usually felt in the stomach region or towards the lower part of the abdomen (usually the entire abdominal region or sometimes on one particular side which may indicate appendicitis). When correctly explained to the physician, the person suffering from the pain will be properly examined for all digestive and organ related issues instead of being simply dismissed as another case of indigestion. A thorough scan of the gallbladder and its ducts is the only way for one to be diagnosed with gallbladder stones.

Arrangements should be made for the removal of the stones immediately because if the gallbladder is left untreated, it will suffer from further bile juice deposits, damage to its tissues, and this will make the pains recurring in higher frequencies in the person. Apart from the pains, chances of cancer setting in become very high and this of course poses a much larger threat than gallstones. At this stage, the quickest solution that is deemed to be sufficient to deal with the problem at its roots is deemed to be the removal of the entire organ.

Another important thing to note is that the digestive system, when emulsifying fat from food, also emulsifies some other important nutrients such as vitamins A, K, D, and E. These nutrients are introduced in the bloodstream via the intestinal lining, and if a sharp dip in these nutrients is observed, then the physician should be prompted to check the body for gallstones formation in addition to reviewing the patient's diet and prescribing food supplements. A regular check-up would be beneficial for a person because gallbladder diseases can be easily spotted in its early stages. Being alert to the various symptoms and being as clear as possible about them to the physician is a crucial responsibility of the patient.

GALLSTONES - THE MAIN CULPRITS

A lot has already been spoken about gallstones, so it's now time to bring them under this book's microscope and examine them thoroughly.

Gallstones' Formation Workflow

So the process, in which gallstones are formed, either in the gallbladder or in the duct, is outlined below:

- *An excess amount of cholesterol is introduced in the body. The excess cholesterol when mixed with bile salts and water forms a sludge-like liquid that doesn't fully get cleared out of the body when the gallbladder contracts and expands to release the bile juice into the small intestine.*

- *When the imbalance becomes too much for the gallbladder to handle or get rid of, there are small crystals formed either within the gallbladder or in the bile duct.*

- *The liver continues to secrete too much of cholesterol in the gallbladder to be mixed with the bile juice but the mixture continues to remain stagnant without being emptied fully.*

- *Bilirubin too can get collected along with the remaining thing and make the cholesterol gallstones turn black.*

- *The stones thus formed over a period of time harden to such an extent that they prevent the gallbladder from functioning properly and to cause an infection in it and the ducts that lead fluids in and out of the gallbladder.*

Inflammation of the gallbladder

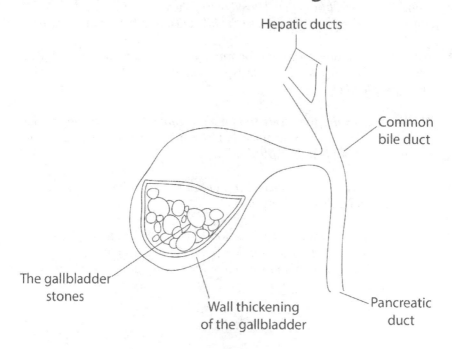

Gallstones, contrary to popular notions, are not found only in the heart of the pear-shaped gallbladder, but can also be found in the Hartmann's pouch, as discussed earlier. As the stone (or stones) block an important passage, they are directly responsible for the inflammation of the gallbladder, the pain, and discomfort one experience. Most people who have problems with their gallbladder are actually suffering from the formation of gallstones.

Gallstones are more popular in countries where people tend to consume very rich food, high in calories, fat, and oil, and do not perform much physical activities. There are not one but several types of gallstones which we will talk about in the following section.

The Types of Gallstones

There are not one but three main types of gallstones! Here are the details about them:

Cholesterol Gallstones

The most typical kind of gallstone, which is found in over 70% of people who are suffering from pain caused by the gallbladder, is known as the **Cholesterol Gallstone**. Out of the total content of the bile juice that is transported by the gallbladder to the small intestine, 5% consists of cholesterol, which has been referred to as fat earlier in this book. As several people know, cholesterol is one of the most important sources of energy for our body, and thus needs to be broken down in the right way and the right amount. The cholesterol that doesn't need to be used is stored in our body, and excess cholesterol deposits make us look fat or lead to health issues, most commonly related to the heart. However, the other organ that can be impacted by poor quality or high quantity consumption of cholesterol is the gallbladder.

Cholesterol in itself is not an easy chemical that can be absorbed by the bloodstream, hence it needs to be combined with bile salts so that it can be emulsified and then absorbed. When cholesterol gets combined with bile juice in improper quantities or in the wrong manner, a thick liquid is formed, similar to sludge. If the imbalance between these two things is much more severe, then from the sludge left behind several crystals are formed. These crystals then get combined to form cholesterol gallstones.

Black Pigment Gallstones

For those suffering from a rare condition called **hemolytic anemia**, the gallstones are usually blackened because of the high content of red blood cells received along with bilirubin. In hemolytic anemia, the red blood cells are broken down much faster than necessary and thus, they also get collected at a high rate without being eliminated from the body. These surplus red blood cells get collected to form stones. The other reason why black gallstones can be formed is cirrhosis (when the liver gets scarred and there is loss of blood under this circumstance too). More about cirrhosis has been discussed later in this book.

Brown Pigment Gallstones

When the cholesterol and calcium levels are very high, they result in formation of stones of this color. It has been found that while black gallstones are more common in Western countries such as USA, a higher number of Asians have been found with brown gallstones. The reason of course is mainly due to the dietary differences in the regions being compared.

Mixed Gallstones

There have been cases reported of people having both kinds of gallstones too.

Note: Pigmented gallstones are usually found within the gallbladder and are thus detected much later than the other type of gallstones. That's because they don't obstruct any passage and thus don't lead to a breakdown of any process. So, the body doesn't send out warning signals in the form of cramps. The process in which these stones are formed is known as **cholithiasis**.

Common Bile Duct Gallstones

These are found in the bile duct or the Hartmann's pouch rather than in the gallbladder itself. This can either happen because the gallbladder stones are moved from within the gallbladder to the duct, or because the stones are formed in the duct itself. The stones which move from the gallbladder to the duct are known as **secondary gallstones** and about 10% of patients who are diagnosed to be suffering from gallstones also have these secondary gallstones present in their body. Those stones that are formed in the duct itself pose a higher infection threat than the secondary gallstones found in the duct, and are thus quite dangerous. The condition which is caused by these alternate types of gallstones is known as **Choledocholithiasis**.

GALLBLADDER DISORDERS THAT DO NOT INVOLVE GALLSTONES

Now that we have read all about gallstones, let us now look at the other issues that may affect a gallbladder, without the presence of any gallstones in the gallbladder or in the bile duct.

Acalculous Gallbladder Diseases

Acalculous gallbladder diseases are those in which a person suffers from the symptoms that are similar to having gallstones but in fact do not have any stones in either the gallbladder or in the bile duct. These issues may be caused due to some catalysts that have been introduced in the body, or sudden actions that have an adverse impact on the gallbladder. They may also be a result of deterioration of other parts of the body over a period of time, usually because of chronic or incurable diseases. Here are the two main types of acalculous gallbladder diseases:

■ If any other part of the body has been afflicted with any chronic or long-term diseases, then this may result in poor or restricted supply of blood to the gallbladder. As we all know, blood is what travels within the whole body carrying a supple of energy factors and nutrients. It is with the help of these that all organs function and survive, barring a few organs such as the brain to which there is no blood supply. So without an adequate supply of blood to it, the gallbladder may become infected, or it may lose the ability to contract and expand as normal. This of course means that it cannot function properly and thus leads to pain and discomfort to the patient.

■ The other issue that can prevent the gallbladder muscles from properly functioning can be muscular issues. It is known as **biliary dyskinesia**. Even the issue of a gallbladder not functioning at the required speed falls under this category.

The acalculous diseases are rare instances which prove that a person may be born with or can develop gallbladder-related diseases, for no fault of his or her. The symptoms may be similar to the conditions that are experienced when a person suffers from gallstones. But the treatment of course should be much different for such patients because there is no blockage that prevents the gallbladder from functioning properly; it is the organ itself or the blood supply to it that needs correction.

3

Identifying Gallbladder Problems

THE SYMPTOMS AND STAGES

We have now gone through the list of the issues a person may face with the gallbladder and an overview of some of the symptoms associated with them. For a layman, it is necessary to know about the symptoms in detail so that one can correctly identify a spasm or a nausea episode to be more than indigestion. When you know that what you are experiencing is more than a regular problem, you will be prompted to seek immediate expert help that will know exactly how to probe you for your illnesses instead of dismissing them lightly.

What should be borne in mind is that symptoms may vary in intensity and duration from person to person because each person is built in a unique way. It is quite possible for a person who has large stones in his gallbladder to have never suffered from any discomfort, but a person who has just 1 or 2 minute stones in his gallbladder may suffer from the most severe reactions. So one should consider all possibilities and not ignore these warning signs based on another person's gallbladder-related attacks or treatments.

Colic, or Biliary Pain

The most common symptom, and the most easily ignored one, is the pain in the chest region, just below the rib cage. This, worryingly, is also one of the mildest symptoms of gallbladder related problems, which means that symptoms experienced in the later stages are only going to be more intense and difficult to bear and deal with. The biliary colic, as it is also known, is felt in the upper abdomen. The biliary colic attack, in addition to pain, has a few other characteristics:

- The pain is steady and gripping. It is felt near the rib cage and in the regions mentioned earlier. It can also move up to the upper back, or can also be felt behind the breast bone.

- Vomiting or the sensation to vomit (nausea) can also be experienced.

- Passing gas, changing positions while lying down or even sitting is not of much help, and over-the-counter medicines such as antacid tablets and powders cannot alleviate the pain in any manner. The pain remains steady and unchanged for the duration that it lasts.

- Biliary colic acids can usually last between 1 to several hours. But if the pain doesn't reduce even after 7-8 hours, then the person may not be suffering from biliary colic but from acute cholecystitis or something much more serious.

- It has been observed that the pain may recur from time to time, say once a week, but its onset is usually around the same time of the day.

- Some people also experience the pain after having an especially rich and fat-laden meal. The effects may not be apparent within a few minutes of having a meal, but they usually become obvious about 3-4 hours after consuming a meal. Some people also are forced to get up in the middle of their sleep because of the uncontrollable pain caused by biliary colic.

- Some patients have had experiences of pains that can occur not once a week or month or even bi-annually, but just once in a few years. So gallstones can take a really long, but quiet time to fully form and become an un-avoidable health concern.

Another important thing that one must remember is that symptoms such as belching, burping, stomach bloating, feeling too full after a meal, a burning sensation behind the breast bone (heartburn), or the sensation of feeling some of the digestive acid rushing back into your food pipe (regurgitation) are not problems that are related to the gallbladder but are wholly related to digestive issues. Some of the digestive problems that may have led to these symptoms are peptic ulcer, indigestion, or gastroesophageal reflux disease. These are felt immediately, or after about an hour or so of consuming a meal.

Timeline of Gallstones' Discovery

- *Gallbladder related symptoms are usually extremely quiet or occur after such long gaps that they are difficult to remember or even categorized as something that you have felt before. It has been found that an average person usually takes about 8 years to realize that he or she may be suffering from gallstones, and that is because while stones are young or in the process of being formed, a person experiences these discomforts.*

- *However, after about 10 years, when the stones have formed, they may cause minor problems. There are just 2% patients who correctly recognize their symptoms to be related to the gallbladder instead of being digestive problems in these first 10 years.*

- *After the initial stages, the body gets acclimatized to the stones and stops throwing warning signs and instead suffers from a major attack brought on by the total inflammation of the gallbladder and its infection.*

Those who suffer from acalculous gallbladder disease suffer from the same symptoms as a person suffering from gallstones or sludge. They also last for a similar duration and can be as sporadic with the others. But the lack of stones shouldn't be taken as a smaller threat.

Acute Cholecystitis

About 3% of the people who have gallstones of any variety suffer from this condition which leads to the inflammation of the gallbladder. The condition of having a blocked gallbladder in itself is known as **acute cholesystitis** and they can be because of both sludge as well as stones. While sludge would be easier to deal with, they pose a no lesser threat than the later and must be dealt with as quickly and efficiently as possible. The symptoms of this condition are similar to that of biliary colic attacks, but they last for a much longer time and are felt more acutely by the patient.

- The pain originates in the same place as mentioned in the above condition (in the upper or right abdomen region) and can also spread to the upper front and back regions of the body. However, the pain in this case doesn't last for just a few hours but lasts for a few days. It is so intense that a person would find it difficult to even draw a deep breath without hurting his or her chest or abdominal regions.

- Pain behind the breast bone or even reaching as high as between the shoulder blades have been reported in these cases.

- People who suffer from acute cholecystitis have additional symptoms of chills and fevers that do not accompany a regular biliary colic attack. The body becomes too weak to function and fight of regular bacteria and virus that it could have dealt with earlier, which is why chills and fever become rampant during these attacks.

- Patients often end up vomiting or feeling nausea on an extreme basis during such attacks.

People who experience all or even any of these symptoms should immediately take medical assistance because the body is no longer able to tolerate the pain and the sludge or stones are posing a large problem that is preventing the body from functioning or even rest in a normal manner. People who ignore such severe attacks run the high risk of suffering from gallbladder gangrene and its perforation (a severe kind of rupture or cut). These of course lead to infection of such high degrees that the organ becomes a threat to other organs. Infection set in about 20% of people suffering from acute cholecystitis. People suffering from diabetes in addition to this condition have the toughest time to heal from such attacks. Diabetes, as we all know, is a condition that is caused because of improper sugar and insulin levels in the body and people suffering from it take an abnormally long time to heal from small cuts or wounds, let alone perforations and gangrene.

Chronic Cholecystitis

Gallbladder diseases that are chronic in nature are made up of two main players – gallstones and mild inflammation. Because of the long-term illness that afflicts the organ, it usually becomes scarred and the muscles become quite stiff, thus making it difficult for them to contract and expand easily.

CHOLECYSTITIS

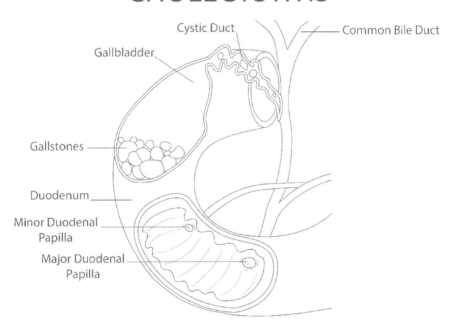

Some of the symptoms of people suffering from this condition are:

■ Nausea, a constant throb (not quite pain but a discomfort) in the abdominal region, and the feeling of fullness because of gas, are some of the most common symptoms associated with this condition.

Although they are not always very pronounced attacks, people who have simple digestive problems too are known to complain of similar issues and thus, it becomes difficult to distinguish this problem from them.

- Chronic diarrhea is the one distinguishable factor that can help people understand that they are not suffering from just poor quality of food or a mal-functioning digestive system. People are known to suffer from at least 4 and up to 10 bowel movements in just a single day for a minimum of three months when they suffer from this condition.

Choledocholithiasis

This is the condition in which the stones are not found inside the gallbladder but are instead found in the bile duct. The symptoms in this condition are quite similar to those that have been listed so far. However, as the stones or the sludge have not yet started blocking any ducts, there are some additional symptoms that can be experienced in this case. They are:

- Yellowish skin (also a symptom of jaundice).

- Stools passed are lighter in color, the urine may be darker, or both symptoms may co-exist.

- A sudden drop in a person's blood pressure because of the improper pumping of the gallbladder, or sudden pickup in the speed of heartbeats because of the excess pressure the heart has to apply to make the organ work.

- Chills, nausea, fever, severe pain in the abdominal region, and vomiting are the most apparent symptoms which should persuade a person to consult a doctor immediately. These symptoms are usually indicative of an infection in the bile duct, which is known as **cholangitis**.

In most cases, there are many immediate treatments that can be offered to the person so that the pain is alleviated and doesn't cause further damage to the other vital organs in the body. The actual treatment for the blockages and infection of course require a longer time and in-depth treatment. These topics are discussed in the next few chapters in this book.

4

The Medical Diagnostics for

Gallbladder Related Issues

So far, generic symptoms have been discussed in the book. Let us now look at the tests and other identification methods used by medical professionals to confirm that the problem is with the gallbladder or its ducts.

ELIMINATING OTHER HEALTH CONCERNS

The first rule observed by physicians is to single out the disease affecting the patient correctly. For illnesses that have common symptoms, it becomes necessary to eliminate the possibility of other illnesses and zero in on the right one. The same approach is used for gallbladder related issues too. Here are some of the illnesses that can be confused with it, and which are eliminated in the identification process:

- **Pancreatitis**

Pancreatitis can be caused because of gallstones. But this form of pancreatitis is different from the pancreatitis that is caused because of other factors. The first can be identified with the elevated levels of pancreatic enzymes which are symptoms of regular pancreatitis. Liver enzyme alanine aminotransferase when found in blood is a clear indication of pancreatitis caused because of the presence of gallstones. CT scans and other lab tests can confirm the presence of these enzymes and the severity of the issue.

- **Acute Appendicitis** – Inflammation of the appendix.

- **Chron's and Colitis Diseases** – Crohn's disease, ulcerative colitis, and other inflammatory bowel diseases.

- **Stomach Ulcers**

- **Pneumonia**

- **Hiatal Hernia**

- **Kidney Stones**

- **Gastroesophageal Reflux**

- **Urinary Tract Infections**

- **Viral Hepatitis**

- **Diverticulosis or Diverticulitis**

- **Heart Attacks**

- **Pregnancy**

PHYSICAL EXAMINATION

The upper right part of the abdomen will always be the most affected region of the person, and the pain will not subside even after a long time. While further tests and scans will be carried out to confirm the diagnosis, the particular spot of pain is a certain indication of this problem. The more experienced physicians or doctors can easily use this method because the pain originates from the same spot always and it radiates to other parts later. People who suffer from this problem will not complain of any tenderness in their abdomen when the doctor presses that region with some pressure.

LABORATORY TESTS

Blood tests must be carried out in all patients who exhibit these symptoms as enzymes and alkalines are the factors that will confirm gallbladder related issues. These can also help a doctor identify if it is a biliary colic attack or a case of chronic cholecystitis.

■ Elevated levels of bilirubin in the bloodstream can be found in lab tests. Yellowish tinge of skin is caused because of bilirubin, which is found in blood and when secreted in excess can be also a problem for the gallbladder.

■ Enzyme alkaline phosphatase, if found in large quantities in the blood, is also an indication of choledocholithiasis (common stones in the bile duct).

■ There are several enzymes whose blood levels are also tested for this purpose, and some of these enzymes are aspartate aminotranferase (AST), alanine aminotranferase (ALT), serum transaminases, and alkaline phosphatase.

■ Those who have a high white blood cells' count are usually suffering from cholecystitis.

IMAGING DIAGNOSTIC METHODS

Abdominal Ultrasonography or Ultrasound is usually carried out to find out what is the main culprit causing the discomfort and this answers questions like: are they stones related? Where are they located? Is it air in the gallbladder? etc. Here are some of the details that can be ascertained from the abdominal ultrasound:

- Stones that can be as small as 2mm in diameter.

- Air present in the gallbladder that is usually an indication or gangrene of the organ.

Some of the things that cannot be identified with ultrasound but are still issues pertinent to the gallbladder are inflammation of the gallbladder without any stones (cholecystitis) and stones that may be present in the bile duct instead of the gallbladder itself.

ENDOSCOPIC ULTRASOUND

This is similar to the above method but the difference is that the device used to perform this function is not used externally but is passed down via a tube through a person's mouth, food pipe, into the stomach. It is then used to capture details from the patient's stomach and other nearby organs, including the gallbladder. The device that captures these details transmits the data up the pipe to the physician and is known to provide a up-close description of a person's anatomy. This method however cannot be used for remedial purposes; one cannot get rid of the stones using the same tube or data capturing device.

COMPUTER TOMOGRAPHY (CT) SCANS

This is especially helpful in identifying the more serious problems with the gallbladder, such as perforation, gangrene, cancer, and common duct stones. Helical (spiral) CT scanning is one of the most advanced technologies that can be used for more accurate, clearer, and detailed data with the use of a low-radiation x-ray tube that revolves around the patient who is made to lie on an examination table.

X-RAYS

There are 2 main ways in which X-rays can be used to identify gallbladder related problems. In the first, oral cholecystography is used, in which a person is asked to consume a harmless pill which contains dye. This dye spreads to all parts of the body, which can make the x-ray possible. In the other option, dye is injected directly into the bile duct and then x-rays are passed over that region of the patient to spot any irregularities.

CHOLESCINTIGRAPHY

This is also known as the **HIDA scan** and **gallbladder radionuclide scan** in many parts of the world. This is a scanning method which is based on nuclear level observation and doesn't involve any invasive methods, such as endoscopy. This method however takes much longer to be completed and has the following steps:

■ Radioactive dye is introduced into a person's nervous system (intravenous) and the material is such that it travels the same path as bile juice.

■ The person is made to lie down on a table and the scanning device moves all over the body. Radioactive gamma rays in the dye are emitted when the bile juice moves from the liver to the gallbladder.

■ The images of the rays that are so collected by the device can take about 2 hours to be made available in a readable format, and there are images captured every 5 to 15 minutes by the scanning device, based on the device quality.

■ If the device fails to pick up any of the dye, it implies that the duct through which bile passes from the liver to the gallbladder is blocked.

This cannot be used on patients who are fasting and consume food intravenously, or those who have chronic alcohol related problems that have damaged their liver to find out about gallstones, and to identify acute cholecystitis.

ENDOSCOPIC RETROGRADE
CHOLANGIOPANCREATOGRAPHY (ERCP)

This last method is also considered to be one of the best methods available because not only can it identify all issues related to the gallbladder, it can also help in getting rid of a few of them, such as gallstones. Some of the other problems that can be treated using this method are biliary dyskinesia and severe cholangitis. This is however an invasive method of identification as well as treatment, and may also cause certain complications, including pancreatitis.

COMMON MEDICAL TREATMENTS

Now that the common medical ways to identify the problems related to the gallbladder have been discussed, let us look at some of the medical treatments prescribed by physicians. This list does not intend to be exhaustive, but contains the options that are most commonly used:

- Oral Antibiotics and Pain Killers are usually provided to people for immediate relief and for people suffering from non-gallstone problems.

- Intravenous painkillers are given to those patients who do suffer from gallbladder related problems and are unable to find any relief from the regular painkillers they have had so far.

- Lithotripsy is the method in which stones have been identified for breakdown purposes. They are usually used on people who do not have other major health complication, who have stones that are less than 2cms in diameter, and who have just 1 or a maximum of 2 stones. Those with severely damaged internal organs, especially in the stomach and chest region, are strictly advised against this option. It involves the breaking down of the stones with the help of laser rays or electric charges.

- Drug treatments – Pills to help with the breakdown of the stones.

- Laparoscopic Cholecystectomy – The removal of the entire organ using laproscopy.

Prior to beginning their treatment process, especially in cases of acute cholesystitis, patients are advised to follow the below steps to get the inflammation of the gallbladder down and make it more amenable to treatments or removal:

- Fasting

- Oxygen Therapy

- Intravenous Fluids' Consumption

- Strong Painkillers except morphine

- Intravenous antibiotics

Dissolution of bile stones can be done in the following ways:

- Oral Dissolution Therapy that involves the usage of pills

- Contact Dissolution Therapy

However, people who seek medical attention because of gallbladder related disorders are often under severe pain and have already suffered severe damages to their gallbladder. So, the usual suggestion is to go under the knife to help the gallbladder become healthy once again. In worst cases, it is recommended because delaying the remediation process by consuming pills can make each passing day a life threat to the patient. Some of the surgeries that are performed on people suffering from gallbladder-related issues are:

- Open cholecystectomy

- Laparoscopic cholecystectomy

- Robot Assisted Surgeries

- Minimal incisions that can give access to the gallbladder or the affected parts and gallstones, if any. This is known as **mini-laparotomy cholecystostomy**.

- Endoscopic Retrograde Cholangiopancreatography (ERCP) with the help of Endoscopic Sphincterotomy (ES).

Some of the explorative methods used to identify the exact nature, location, and severity of the problems are:

- Laparoscopic Exploration and Cholangiography

- Open Common Bile Duct Exploration (Choledocholithotomy)

- Extracorporeal Shock Wave Lithotripsy

- Percutaneous Cholecystostomy

5

Most Common Factors Which cause Gallbladder Related Ailments

Now that we have seen some of the treatment methods that are used for the various kinds of gallbladder ailments, it is now time to look at the factors that are usually linked with them. As always, it is better to know what the causes are of such ailments so that they can be focused upon, and preventive measures can be taken, rather than waiting for the organ to deteriorate to such an extent that is has to be removed and other organs have to suffer because of them too.

The older and weaker a person is, the more difficult it is to treat such issues. Surgeries carried out in elderly patients are always tricky decisions that doctors have to make, keeping in mind the overall health condition of the patient. As mentioned earlier, most of these problems are spotted about 10-12 years from of their onset, so there is a high likelihood that people who are in their advanced years need to undergo treatment for issues related to the gallbladder. As with most treatment options that do not originate from natural cures, there may be complications after treatments are carried out.

So let's take a look at the factors so that we can be more careful in future and avoid those that can be avoided.

■ **Gender**

Women have a higher chance to suffer from gallbladder related issues than men because of two things. First, the female bodies produce a hormone that is known as **estrogen**. This hormone is known to prompt the body to secrete an excess amount of cholesterol in comparison to its secretion in men, from the bloodstream to the bile juice. More cholesterol means a higher chance of cholesterol stones being formed and poor absorption of fat by the body. The second reason is that only women can get pregnant, and pregnancy is also known to trigger gallbladder related ailments. Women who are pregnant should be careful about their diet and lifestyle, and laparoscopy is considered the best way to get rid of the stones that may have formed during pregnancy. But any surgeries for this purposes should be done after the pregnancy term has ended, and not before or during it. It has also been observed that some women get rid of these stones naturally without any medication and surgeries post-delivery, so some time should be allowed to elapse before any medical options are considered.

■ **Hormone Replacement Therapies**

Many women (and even some men) are known to undergo hormone replacement therapies for medical and cosmetic purposes. There are imbalances that may be created because of a high level of estrogen present in the body (which is a hormone that is present in both men and women, incidentally, but in much, much higher levels in women than in men), which would of course mess up the way the body is able to absorb cholesterol. There are chances of not only gallbladder related issues, but even those related to the heart and breast (such as breast cancer) can be multiplied by many folds because of such therapies.

■ **Gallstones in Men**

While it is not uncommon, the occurrence of gallstones in men is much rarer than in women because of the hormonal differences. However, men who do suffer from gallbladder ailments recognize them to be as such quite later in life than women, so they have a more severe reaction to them. They also take a longer time to heal from these issues, have other related complications, and have more severe post-surgical complications than in women.

■ **Gallstones in Children**

Though rare, there have been instances in which children too have suffered because of gallstones. They are mostly brown pigmented stones and can occur equally in young boys as in young girls. Some of the reasons why children may suffer from gallbladder issues are injuries to the spinal cord because of a mishap or accident, sickle-cell anemia, intravenous nutrition for medical reasons, immune system that has been compromised with due to birth defects, diseases such as typhoid, and any abdominal surgeries that may have been carried out in the past for a variety of reasons, including appendicitis.

■ **Ethnicity**

As mentioned earlier, gallstones are mainly caused because of the diet one follows and his or her lifestyle and these are atypical in several parts of the world. While people in Asian and African regions are known to be involved in more manual labor than Hispanics, Europeans, and Americans, their diet too is quite different from their human counterparts. Thus, the people belonging to the latter regions have a higher risk of contracting gallbladder related problems than Africans and Asians. In fact, there are places such as Chile, Peru, etc., who are known to have a high percentage of people who have gallstones for certain during their lifetime. About 80% of all Pima Indians are known to suffer from gallbladder related complications, and almost every woman in Peru and Chile is known to suffer from gallstones. The main factors are not the ethnicity per se, but the lifestyle and diet that is followed in those regions commonly, and the hereditary factor.

■ **Genetics**

Apart from the women in Chile and Peru, genetics is known to afflict people in general for gallbladder related problems. People who have relatives and ancestors (who have suffered from gallbladder related problems) constitute for about 33% of the cases that are reported each year. Some of the ways in which genes play a role in these problems are issues with transport proteins that can be passed down from one generation to another and mutation of the gene ABCG8. However, this factor is yet to be researched fully as these few genetic factors alone cannot lead to the formation of gallstones.

- ■ **Diabetes**

People who suffer from diabetes have a high risk of also suffering from gallbladder related problems, especially infections, as they can be easily contracted and are persistent in their presence. These infections cannot be treated easily and can spread from one organ to another very quickly. The gallbladder related problems in such people, however do not include stones but are mainly inflammatory in nature.

- ■ **Obesity**

An excessive amount of cholesterol that is consumed has to be broken by the gallbladder and this is one of the top causes of gallstones and gallbladder inflammation. Liver produces cholesterol in an above-average quantity and it causes the bile to get supersaturated. This supersaturated bile juice of course turns into sludge, and any remaining cholesterol are let behind as particles that get converted into stones.

- ■ **Weight Changes**

There are people who lose weight very suddenly or those who repeatedly gain and lose weight, almost in a repetitive fashion (known as **weight cycling**). These are just some of the weight fluctuations that can cause gallstones, as the liver is forced to produce more cholesterol along with bile. People who suddenly switch to low-calorie diets stand a 12% higher chance to suffer from gallstones within 8 to 16 weeks of their diet change, and people who undergo gastric bypass surgery stand a 33% chance to contract this problem within 1 year or 18 months after the surgery is completed. People who follow the below diets stand a higher chance to suffer from gallstones and the onset of the problem is quite apparent in them too:

- People who shed more than 24% of their body weight because of dietary and exercise changes.

- People who lose more than 1.5kgs within a week.

- Those who follow a long-term low-fat and low-calorie diet.

These problems are known to afflict both men and women for the same reasons in similar timeframes.

■ **Crohn Diseases**

People who suffer from inflammatory bowel disorder (and irritable bowel syndrome) can also experience the formation of gallstones and the inflammation of the gallbladder, because of the poor absorption capacity of the body of cholesterol and other vital nutrients.

■ **Cirrhosis**

Cirrhosis is usually a precursor to pigmented gallstones.

■ **Organ Transplantation**

Organ transplantation is also known to cause the formation of gallstones. This includes bone marrow transplantations. If the reactions to the transplantations are expected to be quite severe, then it is quite possible for the transplantations to be deferred to the removal of the gallbladder first.

■ **Intravenous Feeding for a Long Duration**

Patients who are forced to nourish their bodies with the help of intravenous liquids stand a higher chance of suffering from gallstones because bile juice is not produced and moved correctly within the body. It has been found that about 40% of patients who have to rely on intravenous feeding have developed gallstones, be it at a medical center or at home.

- **Medications**

  Some of the medicines which are used to control various parts and functions of our body, such as cholesterol production, the density of blood, etc. can interfere with the working of the gallbladder that leads to the formation of gallstones. Some of the known medicines that may lead to this problem are Octreotide, also known as **Sandostatin**, fibrates used to control cholesterol levels, and thiazide diuretics.

- **Bariatric Surgery**

- **Metabolism rate** of a person

- **LDL, High Triglycerides, and Cholesterol Treatments**

  Cholesterol plays a huge role in the formation of gallstones, as has already been covered in this book. The reason is not the presence of high cholesterol in itself, but it is because the level of good cholesterol (HDL cholesterol) may be too low and the levels of triglyceride may be on the higher side. This combination creates a dangerous imbalance that cannot be handled by the liver and gallbladder. Medicines that can cause this imbalance while taking care of some other issues related to cholesterol (such as fibrates – gemfibrozil and fenofibrate) can cause the body to produce excess cholesterol to take care of these imbalances, which in turn leads to gallstones' formation.

- **Blood-related Disorders**

  Chronic hemolytic anemia (which includes sickle cell anemia) has already been mentioned as one of the reasons due to which pigmented gallstones can be formed.

- **Heme**

  A type of iron that is found in some of the foods we consume, heme iron is particularly dangerous when it reaches the gallbladder. Some of the food items that contain a high level of heme iron are seafood and red meat. Some of the foods that are iron rich but don't contain heme iron in high quantities are lentils, grains, and beans.

■ Diet

Last, but not the least, the most important factor that is known to cause issues with the gallbladder, in conjunction with daily stress and our poor life habits, is our diet. The food that we consume plays a vital role in the way we live, the way we look, the way we perform, the way we think, and even the way we sleep! This factor has been discussed in depth in the next few chapters of this book.

Diet plays an important role because it is the main reason why bile juice is produced and it contains nutrients that need to be broken down to be used by the body. Thus, diet, the gallbladder, and gallbladder related issues share an inextricable link. The diet that one must follow to keep gallbladder-related issues at bay, and to keep it controlled, can be found in the next few chapters. There are many things that can be nutritious as well as safe for the gallbladder, and can easily be included in the menu of people who lead a simple or arduous life. The quantities in which food items must be consumed also makes a huge difference, so a week's ideal diet plan has been shared has been given towards the end of the book. People already suffering from gallbladder related issues or who were able to spot the problem in its initial stages and are eager to keep it from becoming more complicated in the future can both benefit from this diet plan.

6

Life after Removal of Gallbladder

Before the book talks about the food items that are good and bad for the gallbladder and what should be eaten for what kind of issues related to the organ, it is important to address the fact that the removal of the gallbladder is considered as one of the easiest, but most necessary, ways to help a patient heal and get out of danger.

WHY GALLBLADDER REMOVAL IS REQUIRED?

Most doctors recommend that their patients have the gallbladder removed because it is an organ that people can live without. In fact, there are several carnivorous animals which survive on fatty foods, and they survive just fine without a gallbladder. The reasons why doctors prefer having the gallbladder removed rather than trying to treat are as follows:

- Gallbladder related issues, whether they are because of gallstones or are acalculous in nature, are detected quite late in the day by which time the organ is usually severely damaged. In order to prevent gangrene from setting in, or spreading if already present, doctors usually prefer removing the organ.

- Tissue-based organs that do not receive adequate amount of blood, or which cannot function properly due to any obstruction usually become inflamed and slowly infectious. These infections can easily pass on to the other vital organs that are close to the infected organ, and that's another reason why gallbladder pose such a threat when disrupted.

- An affected gallbladder when not removed or treated can turn cancerous over a period of time. Treating the gallbladder usually takes a very long time and by then, many other organs may have got infected. Plus, the chances of the organ deteriorating further are highly increased because a person will have to continue to consume food, which the gallbladder will have to continue to try and breakdown with the help of bile juice. This added strain on the gallbladder is definitely not an ideal situation.

- With a gallbladder that doesn't work as expected, the digestive system too takes a huge hit. Food that could have been broken down easily doesn't get broken down as expected which then can also causes issues with the excretory organs.

- Finally, with an impaired digestive system, the rest of the body gets affected on a wide scale. A simple example of one such effect would be the build-up of cholesterol that could not be emulsified properly. Cholesterol, as most of us know, is the primary reason why people suffer from cardiac issues, obesity, break outs on skin, diabetes, hypertension, and a variety of different related problems.

An advanced problem that has affected a whole organ threatens to shut down the complete organ system, one organ after another. It is nearly impossible to repair the root problem well enough to be able to operate on it and prevent the remaining organs from suffering further problems. Thus, removal of the organ is a very common practice followed all around the world.

People who have had their gallbladder removed will of course face some challenges post-surgery, but it has been found that more 90% of the people who have undergone such surgeries are able to lead a normal life with minimal changes to their diet. Those who lead reasonably healthy lives don't have to make big sacrifices either. The major impact is on the kind of food one eats, which has been discussed a little later in this book.

Open cholecystectomy as this procedure is called, is performed in almost all major health institutions. While it is a critical surgery to save a person's life, the complexity of the surgery is not as much as that of a heart or brain surgery. There are a few things that people experience or are asked to be alert to after the surgery has been completed:

■ As the organ has been removed, it is only to be expected that a person will experience some amount of discomfort in the abdominal regions while the surgery wounds and the affected internal regions repair themselves. It is important to avoid all forms of strenuous activities during this period and people should take care to monitor their diets severely for at 3-6 months post-surgery.

■ Doctors advise such patients to stay off carbs and fatty foods as much as possible for at least 4-6 months after the surgery. This is because the organ that acted as the repository for bile juice required to emulsify fat is no longer present and thus, bile may not be stored in the required quantity or fashion to be able to breakdown a good amount of fat. The lower the fat content, the lesser the body will have to work to emulsify it.

■ A missing gallbladder means there is no checkpoint between the liver and the intestine to regulate the release of bile juice from one organ to the other. Therefore, the body will continue to produce bile, but it won't be introduced in the small intestine in the right manner. Food will therefore not be digested as it used to be earlier. So digestion-friendly foods should take top priority in a person's life post-surgery.

■ Another important thing that will happen as a result of hampered digestion is the frequency and ease of bowel movements. Food that cannot be digested well enough is eliminated from our body via the excretory system. With the removal of the gallbladder and the spike in poor digestion of food, the amount of waste that needs to be eliminated (both urine and stool) would also increase. So a person will have to use the washroom with a higher frequency than he/she used to earlier.

- There will be some discomfort felt if a person indulges in a meal that was too rich or fatty. The common symptoms would be stomach aches as the body has to suddenly deal with a large intake of fat. So avoid those rich gravies and meat steaks at a dinner party because while your mind knows it's a special occasion, your stomach doesn't quite know that yet!

GALLBLADDER SURGERY

The surgery itself is quite simple. With the use of anesthesia, the patient is made to relax post which the doctor will make an incision (cut) in the patient's stomach. After carefully pushing aside the skin, flesh, and blood vessels that get exposed, the doctor will reach the gallbladder. The organ is removed carefully. The loose ends left because of the removal are then surgically sewed shut. Thereafter, the initial incision made is also closed after reorganizing the internal parts as neatly as possible. The surgery is then complete and the patient enters the recuperative stage.

DOCTORS' ADVICES TO THEIR PATIENTS

Like with any other surgery, there are a number of rules that a patient must follow post gallbladder removal. Some of the most common ones are:

- The patient is advised to drink plenty of fluids to keep the body well hydrated and functioning as smoothly as possible.

- Doctors will keep you under observation for some time to ensure the wounds that were caused because of the surgery are healing well and there is no infection or excessive bleeding that need to be dealt with.

- People who lift heavy objects during their workouts or during their work are advised not to lift anything heavier than 10 pounds in the first few months post-surgery as there are plenty of internal muscles or tissues that may get damaged in the process.

- General hygiene should be followed at all times, such as keeping the hands clean and as far as possible from the incision areas in the stomach, changing bandages regularly, and wearing comfortable clothes to allow the wounds to heal quickly and as well as possible, are some of the other tips given by doctors.

■ The common tips given to people after a surgery with respect to food are to avoid fatty foods and eat small but regular meals always. Fried foods too are completely banned for people who have had their gallbladder removed.

■ Some people are recommended to take medicines to regulate the production and movement of bile juice in their body. Initially, after a surgery, most people have to rely on such medicines. However, with regular good food habits and diets that contain a lot of fiber and low fats, many people have been successful in completely shaking off all symptoms that are felt after a gallbladder removal surgery. Some people have also been able to lead a very healthy lifestyle without any medication at all, but that is only after they have paid a lot of attention to the diet that they follow and after a few months of the surgery.

After a heavy meal some people feel certain after-effects such as cramps and the urgency to use the bathroom due to increased bowel movements. As the gallbladder plays an important role in the digestion of food, the impact of course is largely felt during the digestion of food. There are a lot of changes that have to be made not just to the kind of food that one must have but also to the timings and frequency with which they must be consumed.

As long as a person follows the important rules related to nourishment and makes healthy changes to his or her lifestyle, it is quite possible for one to enjoy a normal life, performing all the activities that one used to. Read on to know more about food habits that are good for people who want to maintain a healthy gallbladder and overall good health, and those that are recommended for people who have had their gallbladder removed.

7

Life Habits to Prevent a Gallbladder Attack

Problems related to the gallbladder may not be a very common phenomenon in all parts of the world, but the alarming thing is that it is gradually becoming the most prominent one. It is causing discomfort more frequently and is leading to an increased number of deaths each year. In the US alone, it is estimated that approximately half a million gallbladders are removed every year. For a problem that cannot be pinpointed to just one reason, and which cannot be detected in its early stages, it is more important to follow as many healthy steps as possible to avoid the condition. While it is true that the food that we eat plays the most important role in the formation of gallstones and other gallbladder related problems, there are other reasons also that need to be paid attention to.

In a while, the book is going to only focus on food related aspects and their impact on gallbladder. But one should not make the mistake of only relying on food changes to help him or her prevent the problem from being born or worsening, or to help one recover from a gallbladder removal surgery. Thus, there are changes that need to be made to one's lifestyle too. Here are the most important ones:

Healthy Weight Maintenance

While it is necessary to make changes to the food that we eat, the changes should be in accordance with a person's height, weight, profession, and health conditions. Eating a well-balanced meal that cuts down on fats and focusing on the important nutrients one needs to remain active, will go a long way in helping a person maintain an optimum weight. BMI check-ups should not be a part of only those who visit the gym but something that everyone should keep an eye on. The goal is to get to the range that is normal for a person according to his or her height, gender, and age.

Eating Meals

Starvation is not a solution for any problem, and certainly not for gallstones. A surplus production of bile that is not being used to digest any food is bound to irritate an already inflamed or infected gallbladder even further. It will only cause irregularities with digestive functions, worsen the condition of the gallbladder and of other organs too. What's more, eating regular meals will help the entire body's immune system to be in top form. Regular meals that consist of healthy foods help one in avoiding gallbladder related problems, and also cut down on the chances of other problems, which may have an indirect impact on the gallbladder.

Importance should be given on avoiding fatty foods, as excess cholesterol will directly lead to the creation of cholesterol stones that may or may not be pigmented. A well-balanced meal (that has been discussed in detail a little later in the book) that consists of fibre, vegetables, fruits, lean meats, and dairy products that are low-fat should be consumed at regular intervals. By controlling the quantity and quality of food being consumed, one can avoid obesity which has been found to be one of the key reasons of suffering from gallstones.

In addition to eating well balanced meals, the focus should be on cutting back on lengthy periods of avoiding food. Sitting at the office desk or travelling for long periods without any food is a common thing for most people now-a-days. What they don't realise is that the body needs nutrition. And once it is habituated to a particular food routine, it is difficult for the internal organs to adjust to sudden changes in it. So if you are used to eating your lunch at 1PM every day, and you skip your lunch one day, your body of course will perform certain actions that it has to, irrespective of receiving food or not at that time. So the bile juice that was produced to emulsify fat and help in digestion will be produced but it will remain unused in the gallbladder. One must eat regular meals in small quantities so that no bile remains unused in the gallbladder.

Exercising Regularly

When it comes to food and health, it becomes natural to also include exercise in the equation. It is difficult to imagine life that has a lot of healthy food and relaxation but no exercise. There comes a point when all the healthy food cannot stop the body from effects like obesity, skin problems, fatigue, poor immunity, blood circulation, amongst the many other possibilities. It has been found that people who exercise for just 45 minutes a day can reduce the chances of developing gallstones by a huge margin. Exercises that help in burning fat and improve blood circulation were found to be the most effective ones.

Endurance exercises, also known as **cardio exercises**, for about 30 minutes a day help in eliminating the formation of any gallstones and also help with good heart functioning, which means improved pumping of blood to all parts of the organ. With improved blood supply, the chances of the gallbladder, or any other organ for that matter, also diminish by a large extent. Exercising for at least 5 days a week, for an average of one hour every day, should be a must for people of all ages. The level of stress that one puts the body through will of course vary according to one's age and general health condition, but even the people of advanced years should not stop exercising. Simple activities such as a brisk walk of about 45 minutes early in the morning when the air is a little less polluted can work wonders!

Moderate consumption of caffeinated Beverages

Moderate consumption of caffeinated beverages such as coffee and tea is also known to have a marked effect on the formation of gallstones. It has been found that people who drink a cup of coffee and a couple of cups of teas on a regular basis have reduced gallbladder absorption; they can ward off the formation of gallstones. The research has been carried out on humans as well as dogs suffering from gallstones. The dogs were not subjected to any chemical experiments but they were simply fed their regular meals, which contain some amount of cholesterol (just like human diets do). The only difference that was made for testing purposes was the addition of a very small amount of caffeine in the water that they drank. It was proven that the dogs that were fed water with caffeine were able to avert the formation of gallstones as compared to those dogs which were not fed any caffeine.

In addition to eating a good meal, these habits have been known to decrease the chances of formation of gallstones. Issues related to the gallbladder that are caused due to genetic problems, or ones that relate to the muscles of the organ, however, cannot be avoided or controlled. What can be done is eating healthy food so that any problems that may exist with the gallbladder may be controlled and are not allowed to turn into bigger problems related to obesity or blood problems.

Even those who have already had their gallbladder removed can benefit from leading a healthy life by avoiding fatty and deep fried foods. In addition to avoiding such foods, one must also try and avoid consumption of too much alcohol, indulging in narcotics and cigarettes, and any other addictive substance that can impair one's nervous system and leads to an overall slowness in a person's activities.

8

Foods and Habits that Are Best

Avoided For the Gallbladder

While most of the foods that may be unhealthy for the gallbladder can also be categorized as poor for the body in general. There are certain types of foods that are deemed to be more harmful for the gallbladder. In this chapter, we are going to look at the food types that are known to cause gallbladder related problems in the long run, and must be avoided to lead a life that is free from gallbladder and other digestive problems.

The endeavour is to cover all the food items that can prove to be harmful, but the cuisines that are followed all around the world vary a lot. It is important to consult a local physician or a dietician in addition to reading this book because there may be food types that are not included in this book which can actually be harmful for a person's health. Apart from consulting a local dietician for a proper meal plan that suits your nationality and your daily lifestyle, you can also look at the items listed in the good and bad sections of this book to get a general idea of what should be avoided and what can be included. The idea is not to only avoid the listed food items but to avoid the ingredients in them that can be harmful. For example, a slice of pastry that is rich in butter and cream can definitely be harmful for a person suffering from diabetes and gallstones, but a slice of cake that is made of low-fat butter and gluten-free flour without any cream can actually be a healthy snack. So the culprits here are high-fat butter and extra sweet sugar, not the pastry slices themselves.

To make it easy for the readers of this book, here is a ready reference of some of the foods that are considered to be bad for the health for a person who is already suffering from gallbladder related problems. These may be related or un-related to gallstones, so this is a common list that can be used by all patients who are either recovering from a gallbladder removal surgery or those who have been advised to take things easy else they will have to undergo one such surgery.

FOODS TO AVOID

■ **Eggs**

The high content of fat in the yolk of the egg has been known to cause digestive issues for people who suffer from gallbladder related problems and those who want to lose weight. The white of the eggs contains a lot of proteins so that can be consumed quite easily. In fact, people who work out in the gym or just exercise regularly are advised to include a portion of egg whites in their daily diet. But the intake of whole eggs specifically should be avoided by people with gallbladder related issues. These include wholly organic eggs and/or those that have been factory farmed.

■ **Pork**

Pork is another source of a lot of fat and meat textures that is hard to be broken down.

■ **Fowl Meat**

Fowl meat such as turkey and chicken. The ones that are factory farmed are always presumed to pose a bigger risk. They should be avoided for some time by people who have just got out of the hospital after a gallbladder removal surgery. Those who have been diagnosed with any form of gallbladder problem are also advised to stay away from such meat until the organ is healed, so that there is not much pressure applied on the digestive system and the gallbladder to digest food. Meat can be re-introduced in the diet only if required and on very limited basis initially.

- **Dairy Products**

Avoid all forms of dairy products after a surgery and include them only in limited quantities. Only completely fat-free variants should be included if you are suffering from gallbladder problems currently and want to avoid a surgery. Pasteurized milk, butter, cheese, clarified butter (popularly known as **ghee** in some Asian countries and one of the highest sources of fats amongst milk products) should be avoided completely. Some people do not have any issues after consuming raw, unpasteurized milk that is taken fresh from farm animals that have not been subjected to hormonal treatments, but it is hardly possible for everyone to get such fresh, unadulterated milk. Some people also have very less tolerance for milk and all milk based products, including beverages such as coffee and tea, and complain of indigestion and excessive burping after consuming even a cup of these beverages. It is best to avoid dairy products completely to provide the stomach and the gallbladder some respite and let the body build some tolerance for milk and its products before it is re-introduced in the diet on a gradual basis. Even when re-introduced, care should be taken to consume milk that is fresh and that is low-fat.

- **Grains and Gluten based products such as Breads and Cookies**

Products containing grains such as barley, rye, wheat, kamut, and spelt are to be avoided for the large parts and must be consumed in very limited quantities, if they must be included in the meal.

- **Decaf or Regular Coffee**

Yes, the book did refer to drinking some amount of tea or coffee to avoid getting gallstones. But that was a suggestion for people who do not suffer from any gallbladder related diseases and can prevent their onset. People who already suffer from it or are recovering from a surgery performed to get rid of the gallbladder must avoid coffee of all types because they cause an inflamed or infected gallbladder to react further to it. And for those who have had their gallbladders removed – the digestive system finds it harder to make use of such beverages which may lead to further digestive problems.

- **Grapefruits and Oranges**.

- **Nuts**

Nuts such as cashews, walnuts, almonds, etc. as these too contain some amount of cholesterol and are difficult to digest by an impaired digestive system.

- **Vegetable Oils**

Vegetable oils made out of sunflowers, groundnuts, etc.

- **Foods that contain Trans-Fats**

Be sure to read the label of any pre-cooked or packed food items, or ready to cook or eat dishes that you pick up from the supermarket the next time. If they contain trans fats, they should be excluded from your shopping list because trans fats are more difficult to digest than natural fat found in foods that we freshly prepare and consume.

- **Hydrogenated and partly Hydrogenated Oils**.

- **Deep and Shallow Fried foods**

This particular category includes a number of items, but the most common ones that can be listed here are wafers, potato chips, fresh fries, and snacks made out of fried meat.

- **Margarine**

An alternative to oil but not at all healthy, this clogs the arteries faster than regular vegetable based oils do. But even worse, it applies a lot of pressure on the digestive system while being broken down because it contains a high amount of hard to digest fat.

- **Saturated Fat based Foods**.

- **Spicy Foods**

    Your favorite bowl of Chinese vegetable soup that is made out of spicy sauces needs to be replaced with food that doesn't contain spices. Spicy food, even on a normal stomach, causes a lot of acidity, and regular consumption of over-spicy food is generally said to be very bad for health. However, a digestive system that is impaired with a faulty gallbladder, or the lack of one, will find it tougher to handle the spice content of food and this will lead to burning sensations and many other discomforts.

- **Red Meats**

    Such as beef and mutton, as these contain a high amount of fats and are difficult to be digested by a person even in general.

- **Liqueur**

    Alcohol of any kind, be it whiskey, beer, wine, or even cocktails must be avoided at all costs.

- **Turnips**.

- **Carbonated Water (including Cola, Soda, and other Fizzy Drinks)**.

- **Chocolate and chocolate based Products**.

- **Ice Cream**

    As this is primarily made out of milk and milk-based products and also contains a number of additive flavours, artificial colours, and processed food ingredients, any variety of ice cream can cause a person to suffer from digestive problems.

- **Tap water**

  Water that has not been boiled may contain a number of harmful bacteria and other harmful microorganisms that cannot be seen by the naked eye but can wreck havoc if they enter our body. The chances of suffering from further infections and inflammations because of these microorganisms increase by many fold with the consumption of tap water that has not been boiled well.

- **Cauliflower and Cabbages**

  These vegetables are said to be very difficult to digest even by a normal person, or those who suffer from even mild indigestion. Because of the consumption of these vegetables, used in rice, in curries, or in soups most commonly, people are known to develop indigestion and some digestive systems find it tough to even break these items down fully. Moreover, as a result of all the strain that is put on the digestive systems, it is not uncommon for people to let out gas (flatulence) which is loud and smelly, as a side effect. Many people start letting out gas 3-4 hours after consuming a meal containing these vegetables. This problem can persist even until the next day until the body is finally able to fully digest them! So avoiding them after losing the gallbladder or when one is about to lose it is definitely a good idea!

- **Oats**

  Some people suffer from adverse reactions after consuming oats, either with milk or with some spices in the form of a curried porridge, and they should add this grain to the list of grains that must be avoided.

- **Glucose based Products**

  Sugar, artificial sweeteners, preservatives, and jiggery should be avoided as well.

■ **Refined and Bleached Foods**

Food items made out of refined oil, and white flour (which is popularly known as "**maida**" in certain Asian countries) should be avoided as well. Maida, or bleached and refined flour is also made out of wheat, but it is milled and refined to an extra degree because of which its colour and the texture of the foods made with it are quite different from the usual wheat-based products. Refined and bleached white wheat flour is harder for the stomach to digest and hence is best avoided.

■ **Allergic Foods**

Foods to which one is even mildly allergic too should be avoided. Consuming them even in small quantities can trigger an out-of-proportion reaction in people who suffer from gallstones.

■ **Food Dressings**

Don't we all love an extra slice of the pizza that is loaded with feta or Parmesan cheese? Or that topping of whipped cream on top our cold coffee or soft pineapple and strawberry layered cake? Another popular food dressing that seems to be invading even healthy dishes like salads is mayonnaise. Originally to be used as a dip like guacamole, mayonnaise is another dairy-based product that is being increasingly used in a large number of dishes and that should be avoided not only to get rid of gallbladder related problems, but to avoid obesity in general. Food dressings contain a number of artificial sweeteners and loads of calories and add no nutritional value to the foods that we consume and can easily be avoided. The only compromise that will be done would be with the taste-buds, but with an impaired gallbladder, that should be an easy one to make!

When a person has recovered considerably from gallbladder removal surgery, he or she would be advised to slowly acclimatize him/herself with regular foods but still maintain constraints on the quality and quantity of foods being consumed. Foods that are generally bad for health should be avoided altogether, but here is a list of alternate foods that can be consumed by a recovering patient. These are foods that are listed as alternates to the foods that have been mentioned in the "banned" list. Some of the items listed in the "approved" list may feature in the "banned" list above, but you should remember that these should be consumed only in small portions and only after a person has fully recovered from the gallbladder removal surgery. For people who continue to have the gallbladder but have managed to tame the problems associated with it, then the items from the below alternates' list should be selected with extra caution.

Foods Bad for the Gallbladder	Healthy Alternatives (to be used strictly on personal basis and in limited or recommended quantities only)
Lard, butter, ghee (clarified butter), and spreads (cheese spreads, for example)	Dairy products that are low-fat, light spreads, oil sprays instead of teaspoons of oil for cooking, honey, and jams.
Whole milk, full-fat yoghurts, and cream	Semi-skimmed or fully skimmed milk, half-fat crème fraiche, low-fat or fat-free yoghurt, and low-fat evaporated milk.
Full fat cheese varieties such as Brie, Stilton, and Cheddar	Light and soft cheese available naturally such as mozzarella and ricotta in small portions, low-fat Cheddar cheese, light cheeses, and cottage cheese.
Wheat based snacks such as biscuits, cookies, and cakes, pastries, crisps, and nuts (which fall under the dry fruits' category)	Low-fat, un-buttered popcorn, fresh fruits and vegetables, dried fruits, meringues, toasted teacakes, low-fat crisps.
Pies, puddings, custards, and ice creams	Jellies, sugar free jellies, low-fat custards, sorbets, stewed or tinned fruits, low-fat yoghurts, rice puddings made out of semi-skimmed milk.
Sauces and dressings, for example	Light mayonnaise, mustard,

cream based sauces and mayonnaise	lemon juice dressings, fat-free salad dressings, fresh tomatoes based sauces, salsa, balsamic dressings, olive oil, and vinaigrettes.
Meats (especially the fatty and fleshy parts), processed meats (which include corned beef, salami, sausages, bacon, ham, pork, gammon, lamb, mutton, beef mince, beef burgers, fish that have been tinned in oil, and meat pies.	Lean ham, turkey and chicken in very small portions, lean or extra lean beef mince, turkey mince, haddock, Pollock, fish tinned in water or brine, white fish, and red meat from which all fat has been removed.

UNDERSTANDING FATS IN FOOD

Now, some of the readers may be confused by the terms low-fat, light fat, and reduced fat. These may sound very similar but they actually refer to the varying degrees of fat content that food and drinks can contain.

Low-Fat Foods

In the case of low fat products, the amount of fat found in the foods or drinks is just 3g in about 100gms of the food or drink in question.

Reduced-Fat Foods

Reduced fat products should be selected with extra care. These are not products that contain a minimal amount of fat, but it simply means that these food items contain a lesser amount of fat than would have otherwise been found in it. A whole product that contains 100gms of fat, in its reduced fat version would contain only 25gms of fat, so that's a reduction in the fat content by 75%. But the question that needs to be asked and considered carefully is whether the 25% that is present in the food is actually required and healthy? It is a marketing tactic that is quite cleverly used to market products that have a high amount of fat in its natural form. So Cheddar cheese, for example, has an extraordinary amount of fat when bought in its natural form. But in its reduced fat form, it will still contain a level of fat that may not be required or compatible with the body of a person suffering from gallbladder related issues.

Light-Fat Foods

The third category – light fat products, are the ones that have about one-third the normal amount of calories that one would find in a food item in its natural format. However, this is another marketing strategy that is designed to take your attention away from the worrying act that although the number of calories are cut down by two-thirds, the fat content is only cut down by 50% and not correspondingly by 67%! So selecting the products based on their fat labels should be done with knowledge of its normal fat content that and what is there after a certain amount of fat has been eliminated from the product.

PLAYING THE HUNGER GAMES RIGHT!

Now that we have talked about foods that are generally considered unhealthy for the gallbladder and gallstones, let us now look at some of the practical tips one can implement to incorporate as many healthy foods in the menu as possible:

- Buying processed, pre-cooked and packed or tinned food; and foods that that can be cooked easily in the microwave should be avoided as much as possible. Instead, efforts should be made to cook dishes that are healthy, from scratch. This will ensure that you not only eat very clean and healthy food, but it will also contain necessary nutrients that are otherwise lost in the process of packing and processing foods. You also get to choose fresh ingredients which taste better and whose calorie counts you can keep a track of. Another option that can be considered is the usage of items that don't need to be cooked much, or which can even be consumed raw. So vegetables that can be eaten raw, such as tomatoes, carrots, beets, or those which can be lightly stewed and added to a dish or in a soup, such as bell peppers and broccoli, should be added on a larger basis in one's menu.

- Checking products' labels before buying them should be a mandatory activity and not to be done only when one has some time to spare in the food markets. High fat products should be avoided as much as possible. Products that contain 17.5gms or more of fat per 100gms of a food or drink are known to be high-fat products. Generally, foods with fat indicators have this column colored in red, and they can be spotted easily but only if one takes care to read the labels carefully. Try and buy only those foods that contain 3gms or lesser amount of fat for every 100gms of food being bought.

■ Adding a generous portion of pulses and vegetables will work wonders for your body and of course your gallbladder. So if you are going to make a dish that must contain vegetables and meat, say a Bolognese, it could be improved to suit the need of patients by lowering the quantity of the meat being used, and by increasing the amount of vegetables, and mushrooms that can be used. Make the dish delicious by adding kidney beans and other pulses, and mushrooms that have been lightly broiled.

■ Using an oil spray is an important part of all cooking procedures that should be followed by all households that require oil in the recipe. Instead of measuring oil in teaspoons or tablespoons, it should be lightly sprayed in the pan or any other vessel that is being used for cooking the meal. With spraying, the inner surface of the vessel is adequately coated so the food will get cooked in a proper manner. But, the amount of oil being used will actually be much lesser than what would have been used had it been measured out in spoons. Even if you have to measure oil to be used with spoons, then try and measure in tea and not tablespoons. Generally, just one tbsp. of oil is said to suffice the requirements of one person for a day.

■ For those dishes that are made with a lot of oil, or in which all the oil doesn't get used (especially in cases of fried foods), it would be best to rest the fried items on some tissues or absorbent paper so that the excess oil can be soaked by it, and the food becomes as free of oil post-cooking as possible. Just press your finger in the food that is being served, and if you see it being saturated with oil (which will be clearly visible in the form of small oil bubbles that will rise to the surface), then place the food items on a tissues, or press a tissue over them for a few minutes, and then serve them.

■ Apart from considering the quantity of oil, one should also consider the kind of oil being used, and if it really is necessary. Some dishes can easily be cooked and still taste great without the use of any oils.

Rice bran, sesame seeds', and olive oil are great replacements for groundnut based oils that are normally used to cook foods. Another pro tip that can help with health and cooking is that rather than greasing food that is stuck to the bottom of a vessel with oil, it should gently be taken out with the help of a few drops of water.

■ Lime/lemon juice, herbs, dried spices, and low fat yoghurt are great examples of food dressings, and should be used instead of cheese and mayonnaise. Even raw olive oil can be used for salad dressings, so you have plenty of options to choose from in terms of dressing for main course dishes.

■ When meat is being bought, or when it is being cleaned, care should be taken to select those cuts or pieces from which all evidence of visible fat has been carefully removed. Lean meat should be the priority, and skin and fat should be avoided as much as possible, for all kinds of meat-based dishes.

■ Fat tends to settle at the top of several dishes such as stews and casseroles. Generally, people mix the dish well so that what is settled on top as a layer gets mixed with the rest of the dish and it tastes better. However, the top layer of fat should be skimmed off gently instead of being mixed with the rest of the dish. In dishes where the fat travels to the top and can be skimmed off, it becomes easier to remove them and efforts should be made to remove fat whenever possible, because it is not possible to remove fat from all dishes.

■ Another option that people can use to cook food instead of frying is to bake them. Baking, steaming, boiling, roasting, grilling, or barbecuing are great options to avoid oil and to give the food a smoky texture and flavor that will make it more delicious.

■ In addition to changes in the way the food is cooked, changes should also be made to the way people consume foods and drinks. As mentioned earlier, people should try and increase the number of meals without making any changes to the quantity. In fact, even those people who are reducing the quantity of the food must break down their reduced food amounts into small meals that are spread apart by 3-4 hours at the least.

■ When changes are being made to the eating pattern, the other thing that must be observed by gallbladder patients is the reaction that they have to the newly introduced ingredients or dishes in their menu. In the first two weeks, try and include as many of the food items that are possibly required. Observe your body's reaction after you have consumed them. If you do not feel any negative reactions, then it is safe to include them in your meals on a regular basis in future. There are some foods that can throw an instant negative reaction the first time around, but the body can develop a certain amount of tolerance to it over a short period. Try having the same food or beverage after a two weeks' interval. If you are still having a negative reaction, then it is best to avoid that dish altogether in future.

■ The best way to measure if you are getting enough fat in your body is to count the number of calories you eat and restrict yourself by consuming 40 to 50 grams of fat per day, all meals included. In that way, you know your body is getting the required amount of fat to be able to function properly, but you are not going overboard with the fat content.

By making a few changes in the way food is cooked, apart from changing the ingredients, a lot can be achieved. The priority should remain on the quantity of harmful ingredients being used at all time instead of only eliminating oil and meat from the foods. The quality of food being used also makes a difference because foods of inferior quality usually contain a high amount of salts, preservatives, artificial colors or sweeteners, or a high amount of fat. For example, the cuts of meat that contain a lot of fat are usually a little cheaper than those cuts that are perfectly lean and only contain animal tissues without or minimal fat. Cooked foods that contain a high amount of fat are usually pale in appearance and have a stench associated with them. Even if you cannot feel the oil, you should avoid such foods if you find it oily via any other sign. The process of not being able to digest oily foods properly is known as **steatorrhea**, and it is a very common occurrence amongst people who have gallbladder related issues.

9

Foods That Are Healthy For the Gallbladder

Now that we have covered the foods that you should avoid, let's look at putting some nutrition into you and check out the food items that are good for your health. Again, the below list is to be an indicator of the foods that can be consumed, but is not a rulebook. Consulting a dietician to find out the foods that are best for you according to your height, age, gender, occupation, and medical history is always the safest bet. Some of the items listed in this "good" list may not be suitable for you as you may be allergic to it, or you may just not like its taste. The best thing for you to do, however, is to find an alternate food or drink item that has as many of the nutritional values the food item has and the least amount of bad qualities. For example, people with allergy to milk can cut out this item altogether and replace it with soy milk and plenty of other sources of Vitamin D and calcium, the nutrients that keep the bone strong always.

The thumb rule for people with gallstones and gallbladder diseases is to focus on foods that are high in fiber and on keeping themselves well hydrated throughout the day. Based on this rule, let's look at the good guys of diet for you:

- **Beets**

- **Cucumbers**

    Just like our body which is mostly made up of water, this salad vegetable too has a high amount of water and negligible amounts of fats.

- **Fresh Green Beans**

    It is best to consume these beans fresh rather than dried or in any other form. Boil and add them to your fragrant rice or add them as sides to your daily portion of lean meats. There are a number of healthy but delicious ways in which green beans can be introduced in your menu.

- **Okra**

    Also known as **Lady's Fingers**, this green vegetable has a number of nutritional properties and can be consumed either in curries, or lightly fried. There are a number of mild Indian curries that can be made using okra, and you can include them in any other sides that you may prepare along with beans, potatoes, carrots, beets, and other such vegetables.

- **Sweet Potatoes**

    Have them boiled and mashed with a dash of pepper and salt, or add them to your preparation of meat, sweet potatoes can be used in a number of interesting ways and is one of the most nutritious vegetables that you can find but which sadly goes unappreciated because of its flavor. While its flavor is certainly not bad, not many people prefer having a main course that is slightly sweet! However, sweet potatoes can be used in a number of preparations that can take the highlight away from its wetness and let the focus remain on its texture and nutrients.

■ **Avocadoes**

World's best source of fat without bad cholesterol, avocadoes are a must for those people who have cut back on sources of fats of all other kinds. It is vital to remember that the body cannot function without fat. Cutting down on all fat sources in one go is certainly not a good idea because it will certainly lead to sensations of fatigue and disinterest in your new and healthy diet. However, with avocadoes, you can enjoy the buttery smooth texture of the pulp of the fruit and get your required amount of fat to be able to function without adding any of the bad fats to your body. Avocadoes can be consumed raw or used in fruit salads and even in smoothies and other types of juices. The other benefit of this fruit is that it can be found throughout the year.

■ **Vinegar**

All types of vinegars to add flavor to your food and as a food dressing.

■ **Fresh Onions and Garlic**

These ingredients are great to add flavor to any curry or even continental dishes. That combination of pasta, cheese, and finely chopped garlic is mouthwatering indeed! However, care should be taken to consume these foods in their natural form, or to be cut and used in food in as natural form as possible. Some people prefer having them raw to enjoy their full benefits without losing any of them to the cooking process, but many people do not like the pungent taste and lingering smell they leave behind. Also, some people find it difficult to digest them. So using these ingredients as per your digestion and taste preference is important. But do try and include them, even if on a very limited basis, in some of your meals. Raw onions with barbecued meat make for a great combination. Adding very few pieces of finely chopped garlic to your next curry preparation can make it taste fantastic. Amongst its many benefits, these cleansing ingredients are known to be great immunity boosters, but only if had in their natural form. Avoid using the flaked, powdered, or any other processed version of these ingredients because they contain more harmful than beneficial properties.

- **Shallots**

- **Tomatoes**

Another vegetable that can be eaten raw or cooked with your favorite meat or vegetable in sides or curries.

- **Cold Water Fish**

Trout and Salmon are best cold water fish.

- **Lemons**

A few drops of lime juice squeezed in a glass of warm water with just a drop of honey are known to make for a great early morning drink. The drink helps in cleansing the body and getting rid of toxins that are added to the body with the food that you consume. All foods, including the healthy ones, when oxidized by the chemicals in our body let out oxidants which are the direct causes of ageing. With the help of anti-oxidant preparation such as these, one can eliminate a majority of these toxins and stay fresh. People who want to lose weight benefit a lot from this because this drink is also known to help in burning fat and helping on clear their bodies every morning.

- **Grapes**

Grapes of all varieties and fresh grapes' juices.

- **High Fiber Fruits**

Fruits those are rich in fiber such as apples, pears, papayas, and berries of all kinds.

- **Food Dressings**

Replacing the old creamy and unhealthy dressings should no longer be an issue because there are so many other options out there! In addition to lime juice and vinegar, using oils such as olive oil and hemp or flax oils can also be beneficial. They not only taste great, but also contain a lot of healthy fats and negligible amounts of cholesterol.

■ **Vegetable Juices**

Including vegetables as a side to your daily portion of meat, rice, or wheat based products becomes a little tough. It is not easy to pack a box of food for your lunch, and for your dinner for all those who work extra long hours. Moreover, packed food cannot be kept for a really long time outside the fridge, and not everyone has the privilege of being able to work in an environment where these perks are considered as normal. So what's the best solution to this problem? Are there alternatives for the way in which vegetables can be consumed? Do people always have to spend a lot of time in dicing and packing vegetables for their meals? The answer is no – rather than carrying diced vegetables everywhere, you can include a tall glass of vegetable juices, made a little more interesting with the use of a pinch of black salt or pepper, and a few drops of lemon juice, to your daily meal plan. There are a number of healthy vegetable juices that you can try. Juices made of carrots, beets, and cucumbers are the most common ones. However, there are other options too that you can try out, especially with the use of green leafy vegetables, such as spinach. Some people also prefer using swiss chard, dandelion greens, beet greens, and celery in their vegetable juices.

Make salads colorful and even more nutritious with the use of baby greens and healthy vegetable dressings such as broccoli, and avoid using cabbages and peas so that the salad becomes easier to digest.

Some of the tips to help you choose a healthy meal plan are:

■ Five portions of fruits and vegetables, either on their own or with lean meats or egg whites should be the aim for everyone.

■ Starchy carbohydrates instead of fatty ones should be consumed as much as possible to gain energy without piling on calories. People who can have breads, flat breads (rotis), pasta, cereals, and plantains should include more of these rather than relying on fried foods that are made of various types of flours.

- Wholegrain foods are much better than single grain foods because the nutrients of a number of grains can be combined, and people who have problems with gluten can eat grains-based foods without severe reactions.

- Attempts should be made to include low-fat dairy products in the daily diet plan to get the necessary amount of energy without suffering from any allergic reaction. Starting on a gradual basis by adding a small portion of these items in your plan daily is the best way to start. If you think you cannot tolerate any amount of these products, be it skimmed milk, cottage cheese, or any other variant, then it must be discontinued immediately and try and find alternatives for them.

- Replacing cooking oils with healthy variants is something everybody should try. So cut out the butter and clarified butter (ghee) that you may have been having for several years, and try and replace them with oils that have unsaturated fats, such as sunflower and olive oils. Even oils extracted from avocadoes, nuts, and seeds can be useful and a healthy variant, but these usually tend to be on the expensive side.

- Fiber that is found in whole wheat products, pulses, fruits, vegetables, and beans is a must. Fiber is extremely helpful in digesting food and eliminating all waste products from the body in an easy and natural manner.

- Water should be consumed abundantly throughout the day. Have at least 2 liters of water, and in addition, try some herbal teas. This would be a great way to get some caffeine in your body without going overboard with it.

People who are overweight should do their best to try and get into the normal weight range as quickly as possible. However, a sudden weight loss can also trigger the formation of gallstones and worsen an existing condition with them or the gallbladder. It is recommended that people who are obese lose their weight on a steady basis, and the weight loss should not exceed 1 kg every week. The ideal weight loss would be between 0.5 and 1 kg per week until you hit that optimal weight as per your BMI check-up.

10

Ideal Meal Plan for People with Gallbladder Problems

To help you get started with a great diet plan, here is a sample plan that should help you get an idea of what kind of foods and drinks you can have without triggering any further problems with the gallbladder or coping with the loss of one. Following this diet for a week should be able to help you get habituated to enough to make this your daily diet for the long run. Alternating some of the items as per your personal requirement can be done, but be sure that the replacements are healthy options too!

IMMEDIATELY AFTER WAKING UP

Treat yourself with a glass of lukewarm water that has been mixed with just a drop of honey and a few drops of lemon juice. This should boost your metabolism rate and help in flush out the waste and toxins of the previous day from your body.

BREAKFAST

Add fresh fruits and vegetables to your plate in the form of a tossed salad with healthy dressings. Steel cut oats, two egg whites, a glass of juice of a fresh fruit (not the packaged variety or ones with artificial sweeteners and coloring!) and a big glass of water should help you get started for the day with a lot of energy and freshness.

MID-MORNING SNACK

Snack on some fresh fruit juice, a few sticks of chopped vegetables, or a glass of vegetable juice with some low-fat yoghurt.

LUNCH

The ideal lunch plate should contain the following items:

- Vegetable Soup, preferably clear and free of oils.

- Large green salad or one with a lot of fresh vegetables added to it. Make it as colorful as possible and dressed preferably with some lemon juice or canola oil.

- Fresh fruits as dessert

DINNER

You dinner plate can be made interesting and healthy with the following items:

- Fresh salmon.

- A couple of lightly cooked or boiled vegetables.

- Baked yam or long grain brown rice that has been cooked in such a way that the starch has been removed.

- For those who prefer not to have rice, replace it with whole wheat tortillas.

- A glass of red wine, if desired.

DIET FORMATTING WITH FIBER

High fiber diet should be made the king of the diet plan post-discovery of gallstones or gallbladder removal. And it's very easy to follow such a diet because it usually includes ingredients that have other vital nutrients and are quite delicious too. Even your physician would ask you to up your fiber intake because a good amount of fiber is good for digestion and eliminating waste from the body. Looking for a little help in the fiber section? Then here are some examples for you:

- **Split Peas** – Contains 16.3gms of fiber per cup, after being cooked

  An interesting way to include this in your meal plan is to prepare yellow split pea and spinach soup.

- **Lentils** – 15.6gms, per cup and cooked

  Make a healthy snack of lentil and quinoa burgers, with a filling of sautéed mushrooms.

- **Black Beans** – 15gms, per cup and cooked

  Chipotle peppers, sweet potatoes, and black beans combine to make a wonderful stew that can be consumed on its own or with a few loaves of whole wheat brown bread.

- **Lima Beans** – 13.2gms per cup, cooked

  Bacon fat, leeks, and lima beans can be ingredients for a hearty soup that can be enjoyed with people who've had to reduce their meat intake.

■ **Artichokes** – 10.3gms cooked, per cup

Lime, garlic, black pepper combined with artichokes can be very delicious if done right. Some of the other food items rich in fiber are Brussels sprouts, peas, broccoli, pears, raspberries and strawberries.

11

Natural Home Remedies for Gallbladder Pain Relief

G allstones can cause lot of pain and must be attended immediately, when a gallstone obstructs the bile duct, it can cause symptoms like sudden onset of severe pain especially in the right side of the abdomen, back pain, nausea or vomiting, bloating, indigestion, chills and clay-colored stools.

Now that we know what the symptoms and signs of gallstones are, here are some amazing natural and home remedies for gallbladder pain relief. Most of these remedies require ingredients that are readily available in your home, so read all about them below and get rid of those gallbladder disease symptoms fast and safely.

REMEDY 1

Apple Cider Vinegar and Apple Juice

Apple cider vinegar plays a key role in dissolving gallstones and alleviating pain. It stops the liver from making cholesterol that is responsible for forming most common type of gallstones. The malic acid present in the apples assists in softening gallstones and vinegar stops the cholesterol. It also prevents the reappearance of gallstones as well as abates the pain that you get during flare ups. Once you get rid of all gallstones continue eating apples as this will help in removing traces, if you have any.

Steps to follow

- Take a glass of fresh apple juice.
- Take 1 tbsp. of apple cider vinegar.
- Add apple cider vinegar in the glass of apple juice and mix well.
- Drink this once every day.

REMEDY 2

Apple Cider Vinegar and Lemon Juice

Lemons are very rich in pectin. The pectin in lemon juice helps in getting rid of gallbladder pain attributed to stones. In addition to it, the vitamin C in lemon juice makes cholesterol more water soluble which boosts elimination of unwanted material. So lemon juice is another good ingredient for releasing pain of gallstones and helps in quick recovery.

Steps to follow

- Take a glass of warm water.
- Take 2 tsp. of apple cider vinegar.
- Take 1 tsp. of lemon juice.
- Add apple cider vinegar and lemon juice in the glass of warm water and mix well.
- Drink this on an empty stomach every morning.

REMEDY 3

Apple, Beetroot, Olive Oil and Lemon Juice

As discussed earlier, each of the ingredients has its own unique properties that help in cutting down the recurrence of the gallstones and also cleansing it. Having a mixture of all the ingredients is a very beneficial remedy for pain relief and removal of gallstones.

Steps to follow

- Take 1 apple and beetroot each.
- Take 2 tbsp. olive oil.
- Take 1 tsp. fresh lemon juice.
- Grind them both and make a juice.
- Add lemon juice and olive oil to the juice and mix it well.
- Have this mixture once every day.

REMEDY 4

Pear Juice and Honey

Pear juice may be used in a gallbladder cleanse – also known as a liver or gallbladder flush – along with oil and herbs. The idea behind gallbladder cleanses is that these ingredients work to dissolve stones in your gallbladder and expel them through your stool. However it is said that it doesn't have considerable effect on metabolizing cholesterol but there is no harm in taking pear juice.

Steps to follow

- Take 2 tbsp. of honey.
- Take half a glass of hot water.
- Take half a glass of pear juice.
- Add honey and pear juice in the glass of hot water and mix well.
- Drink this juice thrice a day.

REMEDY 5

Dandelion with Honey

Dandelion contains taraxacin compound which helps in bile excretion. It is a very useful herb for treatment of gallstones. It also detoxifies and metabolizes fat accumulated in the liver. It indirectly aids proper functioning of the gallbladder.

Steps to follow

- Take 1 cup of hot water
- Take 1 tsp. of dandelion leaves.
- Take small amount of honey as per taste.
- Place one teaspoon of dried dandelion leaves in a hot water cup.
- Cover the cup and let it steep for few minutes.
- Strain and add honey which is optional.
- Drink this tea twice or thrice a day.

REMEDY 6

Peppermint and Honey

Pepper mint contains a natural compound known as terpene which is said to dissolve gallstones. Apart from this, peppermint is a natural ingredient for digestion and is very useful in relieving gallbladder pains and relaxing spasms.

Steps to follow

- Take 1 cup of hot water
- Take 1 tsp. of peppermint leaves.
- Take small amount of honey as per taste.
- Place one teaspoon of dried/fresh peppermint leaves in a hot water cup.
- Cover the cup and let it steep for few minutes.
- Strain and add honey which is optional.
- Drink this tea twice a day.

REMEDY 7

Turmeric Powder and Honey

Turmeric contains curcumin that helps make the bile in your gallbladder more soluble, and honey has antiseptic properties that can help prevent infection from happening. Thus just like beets turmeric and honey help with thinning the bile.

Steps to follow

- Take 1 tbsp. of honey.
- Take 1 tsp. of turmeric.
- Have this combination once every day.

REMEDY 8

Beetroot, Cucumber and Carrot Juice

Carrots are an excellent source of vitamin C and also considered as the golden juice of healing. Apart from this, beetroot builds up and cleanse your gallbladder and cucumber with its high water content helps in detoxifying. Thus a combination of these ingredients makes a good remedy for gallstones.

Steps to follow

- Take one cucumber.
- Take one beetroot.
- Take four medium sized carrots.
- Extract the juices from all the three veggies and mix them well.
- Drink this juice twice a day.

REMEDY 9

Garlic, Lemon Juice and Olive Oil

Olive oil on a daily basis may reduce the chances of gallstone being formed. Because the olive helps to reduce the levels of cholesterol in blood and gallbladder, it may lower the chances of cholesterol solidifying. Olive oil is rich in antioxidants; it may discourage its formation. The slight acidity in the oil encourages contraction of the gallbladder which, in turn, discourages building of solidifying substances.

Garlic is helpful for lowering the concentration of cholesterol in the bile which may protect against the formation of gallstones.

Steps to follow

- Take 30ml of olive oil.
- Take 30ml of fresh lemon juice.
- Take 5 Gms of garlic paste.
- Make a mixture of garlic, lemon juice and olive oil.
- Have this mixture on an empty stomach every morning.

REMEDY 10

Eat Bitter Fruits

Bitter foods such as gentian roots, Oregon grape roots and dandelion greens are beneficial for people. Bitters in them stimulate the flow of bile in the gallbladder, helping in digest fats.

It has been stated that Oregon grape roots has anti-bacterial, anti-inflammatory, and bile stimulating properties. Also gentian root extract is a fungicide, an immune booster, and possesses anti-inflammatory properties. Its bitter principles stimulate the secretion of both gastric juices and bile.

REMEDY 11

Hot Pack Therapy

Hot water packs help eliminate the pain almost instantly. It is the super-efficient way for soothing and releasing the gallbladder pain. The heat of the water helps sooth the pain.

Steps to follow

- Fill up the pack with the hot water.

- Make sure that the water is not too hot for your skin.
- Place it over your gallbladder with a thin towel underneath to avoid direct contact.
- Keep the pack for around half an hour.

REMEDY 12

Proper Rest and Few Lifestyle Changes

In order to cure gallstones attack naturally, there need to be certain changes in your diet and lifestyles. Here are few tips to follow.

Steps to follow

- Drink as much water as you can.
- Avoid fatty foods and eat smaller meals at regular short intervals.
- Maintain a healthy body weight.
- Avoid rapid weight loss and fad diets.
- Include citrus fruits in your diet.
- Drink coffee, as it increases the flow of bile and thus prevents gallstones.
- Follow an anti-inflammatory diet that supports liver and gallbladder health.
- Be more active and exercise regularly.
- Reconsider taking birth control pills and unnecessary medications.

12

Natural Therapies and Yoga Postures for Gallbladder Pain Relief

INSTANT PAIN RELIEF ACUPRESSURE REMEDIES

The acupressure treatment will help in easing your pain and in gallstone removal. At the time of Gallstone pain pressure should be given in all the points individually for 30 seconds with a finger or any pointless pencil.

Based on the severity of pain you can give pressure once in 3 hours in all the points individually. Pressure should be made one hour before meals or two hours after meals. By doing this it is ensured that you can get instant relief from acute pain occurring because of the Gallbladder stones and will arrest nausea and vomiting.

Acupressure points are highlighted in the following pictures.

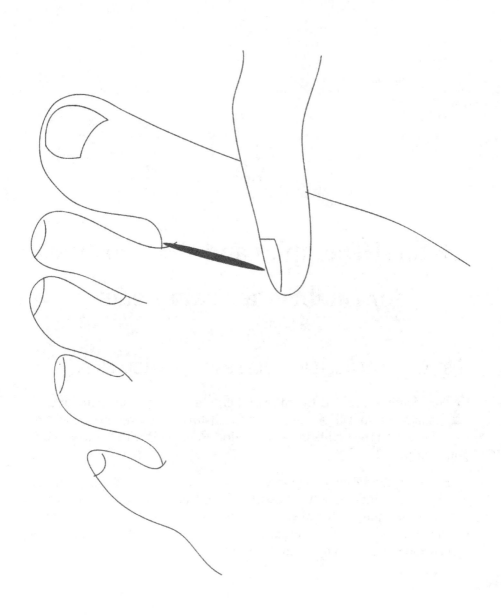

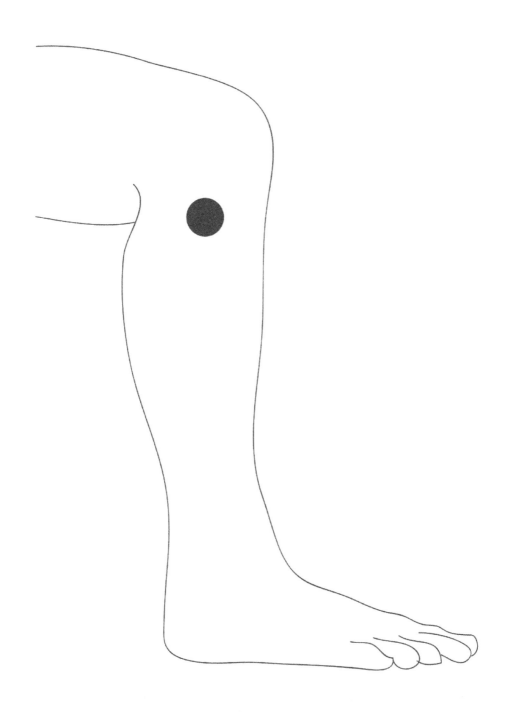

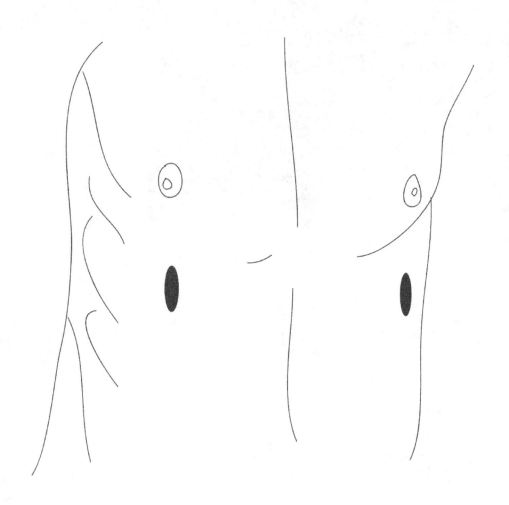

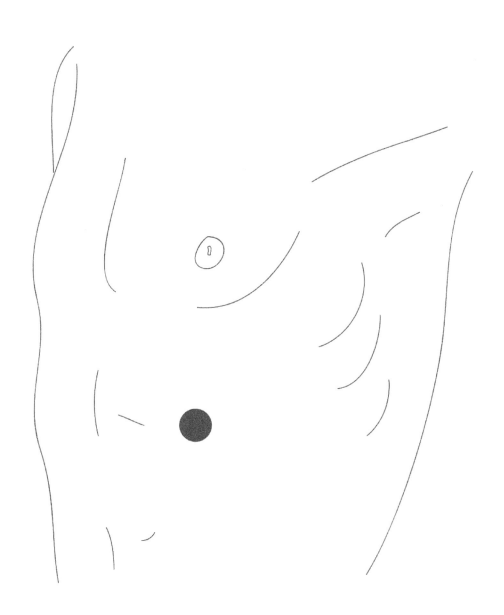

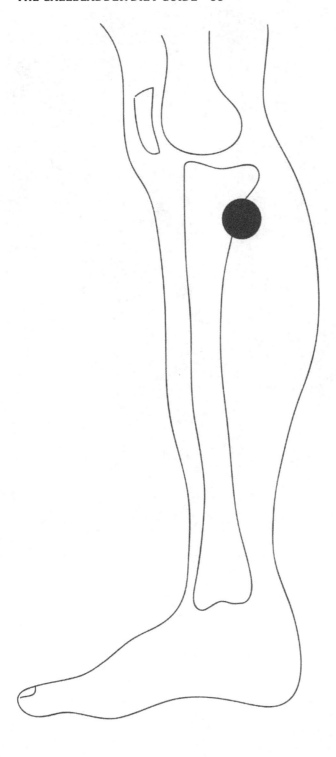

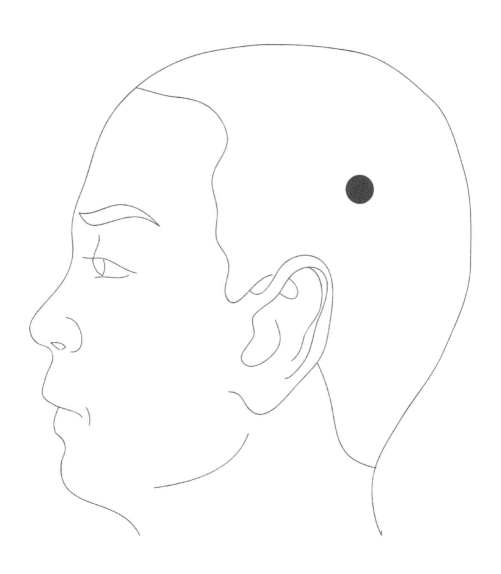

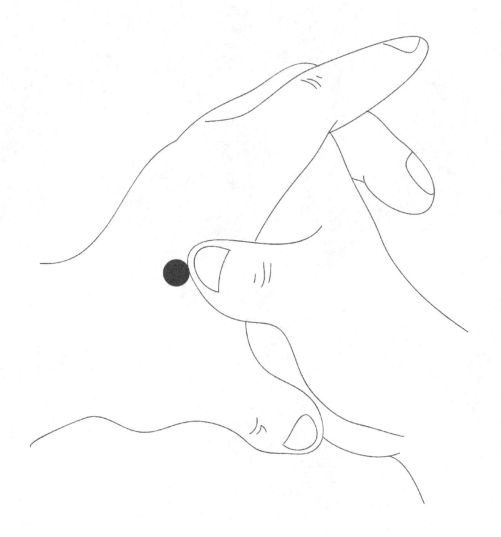

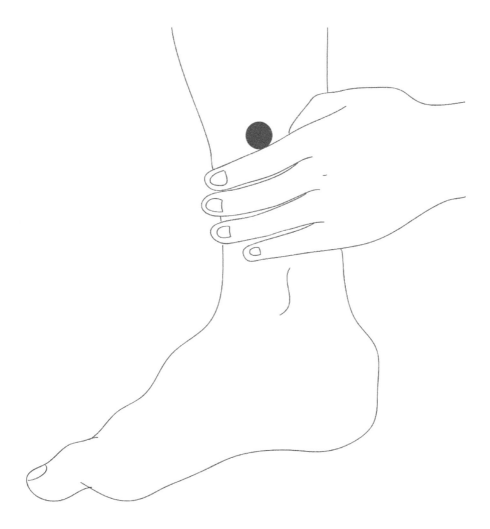

MANIPULATION TO PROMOTE BILE FLOW

Gallstones may block the flow of bile from the gallbladder causing pain or inflammation. They may also migrate from the gallbladder to the bile duct, where they can block the normal flow of bile to the intestine causing jaundice in addition to pain and inflammation. Thus stimulating certain reflex points can help normalize the flow of bile if you have an unhealthy gallbladder. The following techniques help in giving more relief from the pain and it involves the use of a combination of acupuncture meridian points, as well as foot neurolymphatic reflexes. It is adapted from the work of Dr. Bertrand de Jarnette.

The four points you need to know

- Acupuncture point large intestine-4 or LI-4, located in the web of skin between the thumb and index finger on the right hand.
- The reflex point for the small intestine on the bottom of the right foot.
- The edge of the rib cage overlying the gallbladder, which also happens to be the acupuncture alarm point for the gallbladder or GB-24.
- The area where the gallbladder bile duct and the pancreatic bile duct meet before dumping into the small intestine (also called the Ampulla of Vater) is located 1 1/2 in. to the right of the bellybutton and then 3 in. below that.

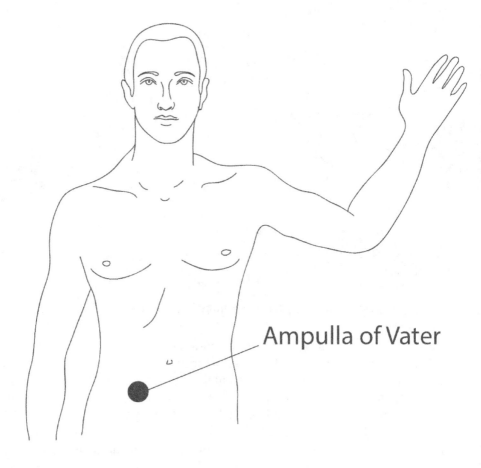

Ampulla of Vater

There are five steps to follow the procedure

■ Grasp the LI-4 point on the patient's right hand between your thumb and index finger and apply a squeezing pressure with a circular-type motion until the pain in the area decreases.

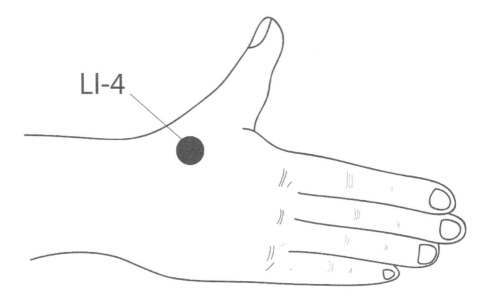

■ Using your thumb rub the bottom of the right foot in a circular motion until the pain begins to subside. (Please see the picture on the next page.)

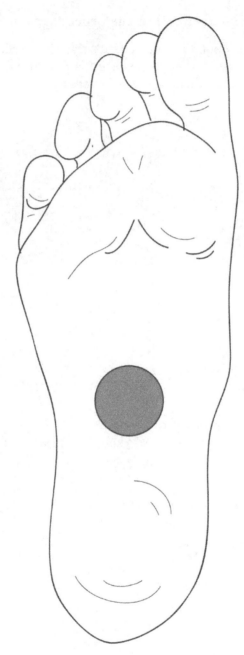

- Cup your right hand so that the ends of your fingers are even and gently contact the bottom edge of the right rib cage. Hold just a slight pressure there for a minute or so to help relax the gallbladder. You may feel a gurgling or emptying of the gallbladder.

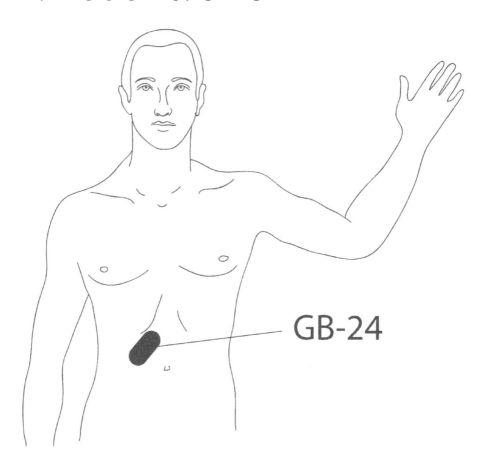

GB-24

- With your left thumb and index finger, again grasp the LI-4 point on the right hand. Place your other index finger over the Ampulla of Vater. Apply about 2lbs. of pressure to each site and hold it for three or four minutes. (Please see the picture on the next page.)

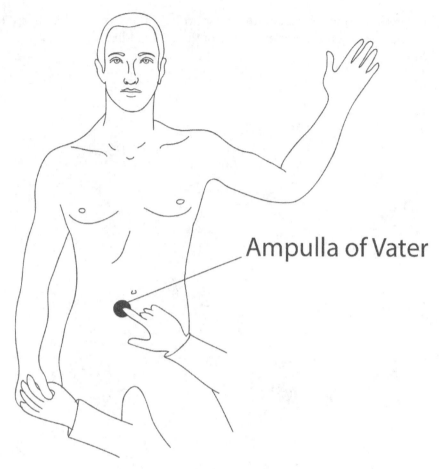

Ampulla of Vater

- Next, apply direct, steady pressure of about 4 lbs. to the reflex point on the bottom of the right foot while at the same time applying 2 lbs. of pressure with your opposite hand to the Ampulla of Vater.

YOGA AND MUDRAS FOR GALLSTONE PAIN RELIEF

Yoga is a well-known technique which brings benefits in regard to certain specific organs of the body such as the gallbladder, by practicing the following yoga poses you can ease the pain caused by gallstones.

Sarvangasana: The Shoulder Stand

It's one of the most effective yoga pose that should be performed regularly in order to get relief from gallstone pains.

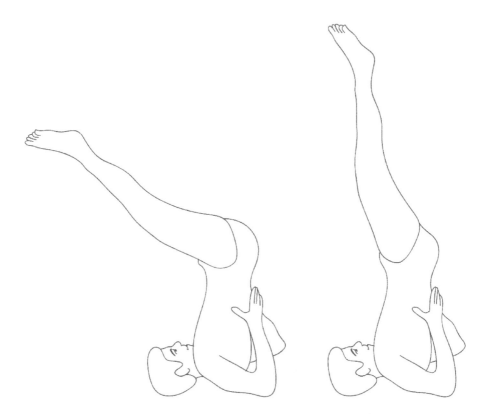

Shoulderstand

Steps required to be followed

- To perform this pose, first lie on your back and keep your hands under your mid-back.
- Then lift your legs and lower body in such a manner that it is supported by your arms, upper back, neck, and head.

- Observe your toes while performing the shoulder stand yoga pose.
- Breathe here for at least 3 deep breaths.
- To come down, slowly lower your back to mat, one vertebra at a time.
- It helps in improving the functioning of gallbladder significantly and aids you get rid of gallstones.

Shalabhasana: The Locust Stand

This pose helps in proper blood circulation. It improves functioning of the gallbladder, activates the enzyme secreting glands and small and large intestines.

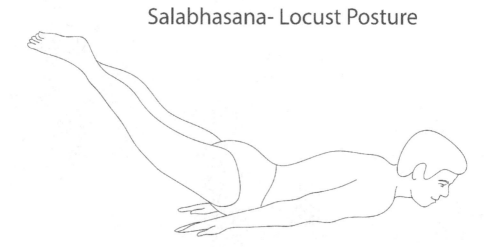

Salabhasana- Locust Posture

Steps required to be followed

- All you have to do is lie on your abdomen on the ground and place your hands by your side.
- As you inhale, lift your legs and upper torso.
- Using your inner thighs, lift your leg upwards without bending your knees.
- Your weight should rest on your lower ribs and abdomen.

- Hold the pose for a minute and then release.
- The locust pose is believed to treat your gallstones substantially.

Dhanurasana: The Bow Stand

This pose strengthens the back, abdominal muscles and helps you with renal disorders as well. It improves the functions of liver, pancreas, small and large intestines.

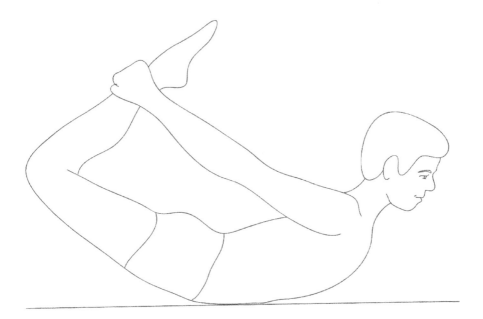

Bow Posture

Steps required to be followed

- To perform this, first of all lie down in prone position.
- Exhale, bend your knees and hold the ankles with hands.
- While inhaling raise the thighs, head and chest as high as you can.
- Try to maintain weight of the body on lower abdomen.

- Join the ankles. Look upward and breathe normally.
- While exhaling, bring down the head and legs up to the knee joint.
- Maintain this position as long as you can hold and slowly come back to the original position.
- The main advantage of this pose is it massages the abdominal organs by pressing them against the floor.

Bhujangasana: The Cobra Position

The prominent advantage of this pose is it tones abdomen, and stimulates the functions of the gallbladder, liver, kidney and pancreas. It improves circulation of blood and oxygen, especially throughout the spinal and pelvic regions and is also effective on uterine disorders.

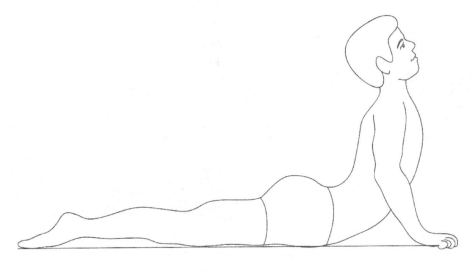

Cobra Posture

Steps required to be followed

- To perform this step lie down on your stomach and feel relax.
- Stretch and join the legs so that knees of both the legs touch each other.

- Place the palm near the chest facing the ground.
- Take a deep breath and lift your upper body like head, neck, shoulders, and chest upwards.
- Keep in mind that elbow should be straight. In this position all weights of the upper body will come on your hands and thighs.
- Here yours inhaling and exhaling plays an important role. So now try to move your head back as much as you can.
- Stretch as much as you can but don't overdo or overstrain.
- Hold your breath for some time in this position. Now exhale slowly and bring your stomach, chest, shoulder and head to the ground.
- Try out this pose and notice the changes in your health.

Pachimotasana: The Back-Stretching Pose

The benefits of this pose are that it reduces the fatty deposits in the abdomen. Disease of the intestines such as Bacterial infection in intestines, blockage in small intestine and more will get cured. Signs of pancreas problems, symptoms of gallbladder disease, causes of kidney stones and Masculinity problems get solved.

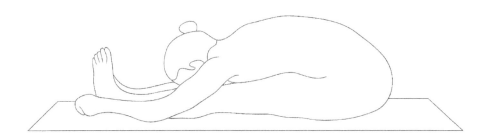

Steps required to be followed

- In order to perform this step, first sit on the floor with straighten both the legs. Bend frontward to catch feet thumbs by your hand.
- Bend your hand knee, which touch on your leg knee.
- Now slowly try to touch your forehead on your knee.
- Don't bend your leg knee. It should lie on the ground.

- Maintain this pose for 30 seconds and simultaneously inhale and exhale deeply.

Viparitakarani: The Upside Down

This pose helps in reducing inflammation and soreness in the abdominal area and also improves urinary disorders.

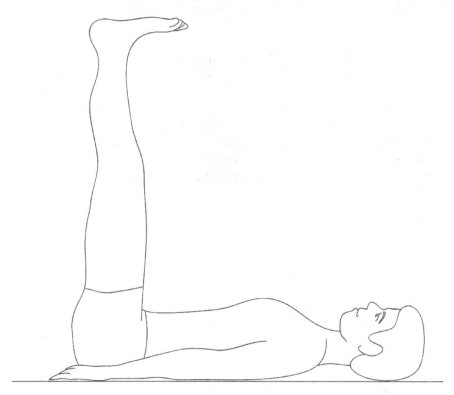

Plough Posture

Steps required to be followed

- To perform this pose start by collecting the items you will need for this session, which ideally includes a yoga mat, yoga block, and two small towels.

- Lie on the floor near a wall and practice deep, steady breathing.
- Exhale and swing your legs up onto the wall so that your heels and sitting bones are supported against it.
- If you have any discomfort in your lower back, adjust your body slightly back from the wall so that your sitting bones are not touching it.
- Rest your head on the mat or floor, keeping your spine straight, and bend your knees a little so your kneecaps won't lock.
- This pose is performed in the passive manner and while practicing it, breathe consciously throughout.

Trikonasana: The Triangle Pose

This pose helps in giving strength to the thighs, calves, buttocks and the abdominal organs. (Please see the picture on the next page.)

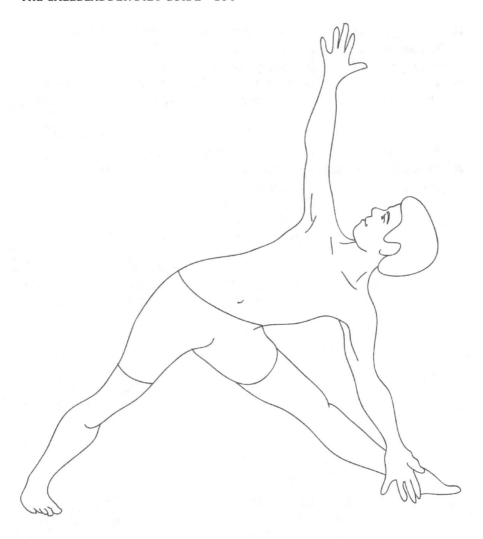

Steps required to be followed

- Stand erect.
- Now, keep a distance between your legs of about 3 to 4 feet's. Extend your arms at the shoulder level.
- Inhale and raise your right arm by the side of your head.
- Now, bend your right arm with exhaling towards the left side by keeping your body weight equally on both the feet.
- You should ensure that the right arm is at 90 degree to the ground (as shown in the picture).

- Maintain the position as per your comfort with normal breathing and come to the original position by inhaling.
- Do the same procedure with the left arm. Perform three to five rounds of trikonasana.

These were the few yoga steps that will help you give great relief from pain caused due to gallstones and also help reducing it. So regularly following these steps will help you stay in a good health.

MUDRAS

Apart from performing the yoga, acupressure or acupuncture treatments exercising with the hands also now as mudras are very beneficial therapies that can be performed on order to ease the pain.

The **Apan mudra** is one of the mudra which sole solves the gallbladder problems. It also removes waste products and releases toxic substances. In order to perform this mudra place tips of the thumb, middle finger and the ring finger together in each hand. Do it for both hands and you will find a notable change if done regularly.

The **Matangi mudra** is another such mudra wherein all the functions of the gallbladder, liver, pancreas are stimulated properly. It is exercised with folding hand in front of the solar plexus or stomach area. Both the middle fingers are place against each other. Note that the attention should be directed towards the breath in the solar plexus or stomach while doing this mudra.

The **Usha mudra** is another such mudra which facilitates endorphin release, a sense of wellbeing in the abdomen, increases immunity; helpful with cancer. All you have to do is for women with palms up, interlace the fingers with the left thumb above the right; gently press down with the left thumb on the right. For men with palms up, interlace the fingers with the right thumb above the left; gently press down with the right thumb on the left.

13

Natural Gallbladder Detox and Gallstone Flush

Liver is the most important internal organ. It must produce an amount of bile that can maintain a good and healthy digestive system and efficiently send the nutrients to all the cells of your body. The gallbladder helps in storing the bile and regulating its flow but the gallstones are clogging up both the gallbladder and liver and in turn preventing free bile flow. Thus a need of gallstone flush arises .Here are few reasons for why gallstones flush and what are its benefits.

Reasons

- Liver's function is to deactivate hormones, alcohol and recreational or medicinal drugs, it filters the blood and provides proper blood flow but the presence of gallstones is preventing the liver's ability to detoxify external and internally generate harmful toxins in the blood. So if the gallstones are flushed then only both gallbladder and liver can function properly.

- The gallstones flush help avoiding the gallbladder surgery because every organ has its own functions and benefits. If the organ is removed it may disturb the functioning of whole system thus instead of removal of the gallbladder gallstone flushing is more preferable.

- Cholesterol lowering drugs lowers the cholesterol which means that bile formed is not proper and it increases the accumulation of gallstones, in turn preventing you from metabolizing fats and removing harmful toxins from body.

- Improper and insufficient fat metabolism is far greater factor in bone density problems than not eating enough calcium. Cleansing your liver and gallbladder will protect your bones.

- The liver regulates hormones and gallstones in the liver interfere with hormonal activities causing hormonal disturbances.

- Many people suffer from skin diseases such as acne eczema and psoriasis if they have gallstones in their liver. Restoration of healthy skin can be achieved through cleansing the liver and gallstones, avoiding the need for dangerous medicines such as Roaccutane or immune system lowering antibiotics.

- A gallbladder with gallstones is preventing free flowing bile and this may be underlying cause of any constipation problem. Thereby resolving constipation.

- Gallstones in the liver are preventing the hormones oestrogen and aldosterone from being broken down and detoxified. These hormones regulate water balance. Water retention is actually the biggest problem for overweight people, far more than body fat. Removing these gallbladder stones will rebalance weight through the balancing of salt and water in the body.

- Free flowing bile will metabolize and break down fat. No more floating stools! Gallstones prevent the liver from delivering the proper amounts of nutrients and energy to the right places in your body at the right time. A clean liver will burn fat as it efficiently distributes fuel to all the cells of your body.

Benefits

- Eliminating gallstones can give you a healthy skin and free from ailments system.

- Liver will be more functional and clear for allowing energy to flow freely.

- It supports whole body detox making the liver remove toxins.

- Helps in maintaining body balance and weight.

- Cleansing of gallstones can give you proper immune system and also proper function of the abdominal organs.

- Lastly you get major relief from the pains caused by the gallstones and the liver stones.

METHOD FOR PERFORMING GALLBLADDER FLUSH

Now that you know what the need of doing gallstone flush is and the benefits of doing it, the following is the method for performing the gallbladder flush.

This method requires one week of time for the process to complete, starting from Monday and completing it on Sunday. You can start on any of the weekdays if you want considering the remaining days making a week.

The material required for carrying out this process are the following:

- Apple juice or cider (real substance without any mixed substances like sugars).

- Citrus fruits (juices as well as whole).

- Olive oil (unrefined).

- Standard Process Disodium Phosphate Capsules.

- Lemon juice.

Follow these instructions from the first day of the course:

- First of all drink as much as apple juice from the first day along with the regular meals till the second last day of the schedule that is if you start on Monday drink apple juice as much as you can till Saturday afternoon.

- Then on Saturday afternoon have a healthy and a normal lunch. Then three hours later at around 3 p.m. take first serving i.e. 3 capsules of disodium phosphate with 8 ounces of water.

- At around 5 p.m. that is two hours later again take the second serving i.e. 3 capsules of disodium phosphate with 8 ounces of water.

- In the evening take few citrus fruits or juices or can have grape fruit or its juice.

- At bedtime take half a cup of unrefined olive oil followed by a small glass of grapefruit juice, or half a cup of warm, unrefined olive oil blended with half a cup of lemon juice.

- After following the previous step immediately go to bed and lie on your right side with your right knee pulled up close to your chest this has to be done at least for half an hour.

- Then next in the morning one hour before the breakfast take another serving that is the third serving (3 capsules) of disodium phosphate with 8 ounces of water.

- Next continue with the normal diet and routine.

During or after effects of the flushing

- If there is any kind of disturbance or discomfort in the region where your gallbladder is located that is the right side of the abdomen just below the rib cages depicts that the gallbladder is being stimulated.

- People will also feel nauseated after drinking the olive oil and citrus juice mixture which is a normal sign and will soon be gone.

- On last day of the course there will be change in the nature of the bowel movement which is the result of the increased amount of bile released after the flush.

- Lastly small marble like smooth structures which are green in color appears in the stool. These are the gallstones that have not yet calcified. This is an indication that the gallbladder flush method was effective.

METHOD FOR PERFORMING DAILY GALLBLADDER FLUSH

This method involves preparing a drink which is especially made for flushing the gallstones and consuming it. In order to prepare this drink, following materials are required.

The materials required for preparing the drink are as follows:

- One tbsp. cold-pressed, unrefined extra virgin olive oil (15ml)
- One organic, unwaxed lemon
- Half pint (10 fl.oz/300ml) of room temperature spring or filtered tap water.

Follow these instructions

- Take the lemon and cut it into small pieces with rind included. Make sure that there are no dark stains or rotten parts to the lemon.
- Now add water and olive oil to the lemon and place it in the blender. Blitz for sixty seconds of time.
- Strain the mixture and have the drink.

Drink this juice daily in the morning on the empty stomach or an hour before the breakfast. Remember to drink this in one go without any intervals or sips. This ensures the flushing and the detoxing of the gallbladder and liver stones. Apart from this the drink restores the pH of your saliva, which in turn helps in absorbing the nutrients from the food taken.

LIFELONG HOME REMEDIES TO PREVENT GALLSTONES

To trigger a more effective solution of cleansing out gallbladder or preventing of gallstones here are few remedies that you can follow:-

Remedy 1

Black seed oil

It is one of the most beneficial herbs and is considered as the best homemade treatment for the removal of gallstones. This herb helps in strengthening the body and to heal on its own. This herb is extracted from the seeds of black cumin which originates in southwest Asia.

Steps to follow

- Take 250 gms. honey
- Take 250 gms. ground black seed.
- Take 1 tsp. black seed oil.
- Take half a cup of warm water.
- Make a mixture of honey, seeds and oil.
- Add the mixture to the warm water.
- Have this remedy every morning on empty stomach.

Remedy 2

Turmeric

The main compound curcumin in turmeric improves the solubility of bile, making bile and its compounds including those that form gallstones, easier to dissolve. The ingredient is believed to be antioxidant and anti-inflammatory.

Steps to follow

- Take half a teaspoon of turmeric.
- Daily intake of turmeric can dissolve as many as 80% of gallstones.

Remedy 3

Lecithin

It is another herb that can be taken for gallstone removal. It is also present in the form of capsules and can be taken anytime.

Steps to follow

- Take two or three tbsp. of lecithin daily.
- Lecithin can be taken with molasses or any other dairy product in small proportion.

Remedy 4

Milk Thistle

Many components present in milk thistle help the liver to function properly thereby making the gallbladder more functional. The seed of the milk thistle contains silymarin, a flavonoid that cures gallstones. Silymarin helps the gallbladder in breaking down the components that can lead to gallstones. It helps the gallbladder with the production of bile which is important mechanism for free flow of the energy.

Remedy 5

Psyllium (Ispaghula)

It prevents constipation, a condition associated with increased gallstone formation. The fiber in psyllium binds to the cholesterol in bile and helps prevent formation of gallstones. It also promotes bowel movements which reduces the risk of gallstones.

DAILY LIFESTYLE CHANGES

To help prevent gallstones formation few daily routine changes needed to be made are:-

■ Increase water intake, drink as much water as you can, at-least 8-6 glasses of water per day.

■ Include vegetables in your diet as much as you can especially the veggies that contain proteins in them.

■ Foods that contains fatty acids, fried foods especially the ones that are deeply fried should be avoided.

■ Stop taking all the products containing white sugar, white flour and saturated fats.

■ Try eating foods which contains unrefined carbohydrates, whole grains and plenty of dietary fibers.

■ Avoid coffee and ice-cold foods and drinks.

■ Avoid skipping meals especially breakfast; make sure you have your breakfast on time in the morning.

■ Also include citrus fruits and foods in your diet for better results.

Wrapping Up!

The original plan for people who had a heavy breakfast, such as lumberjack breakfast, was to follow that up with an arduous day at work, which is why they had to have such a heavy meal. Such meals did not make an iota of difference to their gallbladder because the strenuous physical activities that they performed required the high amount of fat that they consumed, so there was no question of any excess fat being left over, or the muscles of the gallbladder not being worked right enough. The problem arose when the tastes of people remained the same but their daily lifestyle switched from a physically-heavy one to one that required them to sit in air-conditioned rooms in front of computers and projectors for a long period of time.

These and several other factors have contributed to increase in the formation of gallstones and other gallbladder related diseases. The number of deaths due to this problem is low because if caught at the right time and if the organ has been removed in the right way; the body can heal and survive without the organ. But the alarming rate at which the organ is being removed is a clear indication of the deteriorating health choices of people all over the world.

It is easier for people who know how to cook and have the necessary equipment to cook at home to keep their diet under control. However, the problem arises when a person has to rely on outside food for the most part of their lives. Such problems are mainly caused because of the cheap or greasy alternatives that have been introduced to replace healthy and wholesome foods. In addition to the food habits, making changes to other life habits, such as smoking, drinking, staying up late at night, not drinking enough water because one forgot it amidst the pressures of professions can make a lot of difference to a person's life. Removal of gallstones is not the end of the problem; people who are lucky enough to catch the problem in its initial stages should take care to try and improve their meals and daily lifestyle so that the gallbladder can heal and it need not be eliminated entirely. However, for those whom it's too late, it's never too late to make life healthy, and even after removal of the gallbladder; a perfectly full and healthy life can be led, albeit with some restrictions and conditions.

Governments of several countries have agencies which publish reports related to several diseases. It is disheartening to see the numbers which now features in the reports related to gallstones. In USA alone, out of a population of 30,000,000, approximately 750,000 had to have their gallstones removed about a decade ago. These numbers have certainly increased considerably since then. The mean age of people who have had to undergo this surgery was found to be 57 years. Thus, it is evident that people must start taking preventive measures right from their twenties and thirties if they want to avoid any gallbladder related problem later in their lives. There is increased awareness about such problems, thanks to the in-depth research that has been carried out by governments of several countries, but all remedial and preventive deeds start at home, and the key to tackling gallbladder problems are no different. A few changes at the dinner table or on your snack plate can go a long way in changing what your life would be after you've retired and need to reap benefits of your hard work, in a fun way!

At last, I would like to thank you for reading this book and hope that you will create a new healthier you!

CPSIA information can be obtained
at www.ICGtesting.com
Printed in the USA
LVHW080713281018
595065LV00004B/31/P

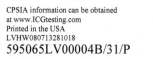

9 781544 174372